DASH DIET COOKBOOK

Weight Loss Plan With Dash Diet Recipes

(How to Use the Dash Diet to Lower High Blood Pressure)

Miguel Montoya

Published by Alex Howard

© Miguel Montoya

All Rights Reserved

Dash Diet Cookbook: Weight Loss Plan With Dash Diet Recipes (How to Use the Dash Diet to Lower High Blood Pressure)

ISBN 978-1-990169-60-1

All rights reserved. No part of this guide may be reproduced in any form without permission in writing from the publisher except in the case of brief quotations embodied in critical articles or reviews.

Legal & Disclaimer

The information contained in this book is not designed to replace or take the place of any form of medicine or professional medical advice. The information in this book has been provided for educational and entertainment purposes only.

The information contained in this book has been compiled from sources deemed reliable, and it is accurate to the best of the Author's knowledge; however, the Author cannot guarantee its accuracy and validity and cannot be held liable for any errors or omissions. Changes are periodically made to this book. You must consult your doctor or get professional medical advice before using any of the suggested remedies, techniques, or information in this book.

Table of contents

PART 1 1

INTRODUCTION 2

FOODS YOU CAN EAT 3
FOODS YOU SHOULD CONSUME MODERATELY 3
HEALTH BENEFITS OF THE DASH DIET 3
CONS OF THE DASH DIET 4
BREAKFAST 5
BANANA AND PEANUT BUTTER SMOOTHIE 5
BLUEBERRY AND BANANA BREAKFAST MUFFINS 6
A BREAKFAST CASSEROLE 8
CHEDDAR, KALE AND PEPPER FRITTATA 9
CHOCOLATE SMOOTHIE 11
FRENCH CINNAMON TOAST 12
COTTAGE CHEESE PANCAKES 13
GRANOLA BARS 15
OATMEAL BREAKFAST IN A JAR 16
PINEAPPLE SMOOTHIE 17
WALNUT AND HONEY OATS IN A JAR 18
SCRAMBLED EGGS WITH SPINACH AND MUSHROOMS 19
SWEET POTATO WAFFLES WITH HONEY AND BLUEBERRY SYRUP 20
VEGETABLE MUFFINS 22

LUNCH 23

BAKED ZUCCHINI & CHEESE 23
GUACAMOLE BEAN CAKES 25
BEEF SAUTÉED WITH ASPARAGUS 27
CHICKEN BURRITOS 28
CHICKEN NOODLE SOUP 30
GREEK SALAD 31
LEMON COD WITH CAPERS 33
GOAT CHEESE AND PEPPER FRITTATA 35
PRIMAVERA PASTA 36
ROAST CHICKEN WITH GRAVY 38

Salmon Chowder 40
Sloppy Joe Sandwiches 41
Tuna Fish Salad 43
Vegetable & Pasta Soup 44

DINNER 45

Baked Chicken with Rice 45
Baked Asian Marinated Salmon 47
Beef Brisket 49
Beef Stroganoff 51
Curried Pork Tenderloin 53
Spicy Pork Medallions 55
Chicken with a Honey Crust 57
Lasagna 58
N.Y. Strip Steak with Whiskey Sauce 60
Pasta with Tomatoes, Asparagus and Goat Cheese 62
Shepherd's Pie 64
Shrimp Kebab 66
Roasted Lemons and Swordfish 67
Turkey and Broccoli Crepe 68

DESSERTS 69

Apple Tart 69
Banana & Berry Ice cream 71
Carrot Cake Cookies 72
Carrot Raisin Tea Bread 74
Chocolate Cake 76
Fig Bars 78
Fruitcake 80
Milk Chocolate Pudding 82
Mint & Chocolate Brownies 83
Oatmeal Chocolate Chip Cookies 85
Parfait Americana 87
Peach Crumble 88
Pumpkin Pie 89
Strawberry Cheesecake 90

SIDE DISHES ... 91

- Baked Zucchini with Cheese ... 91
- Broccoli with Lemon ... 93
- Butternut Squash Fries ... 94
- Edamame Salad ... 95
- Cauliflower Mashed Potatoes ... 97
- Lemon Rice with Raisins & Almonds ... 98
- Minted Carrots ... 100
- Quinoa Peppers ... 101
- Green Beans, Roasted ... 103
- Sautéed Corn ... 104
- Fried Endive ... 105
- Sweet Potatoes & Bananas ... 106
- Warm Coleslaw ... 108

EXTRAS: CHIPS, DIPS AND MORE ... 110

- Dash Artichoke Dip ... 110
- Bean Hummus ... 111
- Cornmeal Muffins ... 112
- Potato Skins ... 113
- Guacamole & Beans ... 114
- Brown Bread (Irish) ... 115
- Kale Chips ... 117
- Sweet Potato Chips ... 118
- Spicy Tortilla Chips ... 119
- Dash Vegetable Salsa ... 120
- Bean Dip ... 121
- Dash Whole Wheat Pretzels ... 122
- Dash Zucchini Bread ... 124
- Zucchini Parmesan Chips ... 126

PART 2 ... 128

INTRODUCTION ... 129

CHAPTER 1: THE DASH DIET BASICS: LOWERING BLOOD PRESSURE AND LOSING WEIGHT ... 131

HIGH BLOOD PRESSURE AND THE DASH DIET SOLUTION 133
THE DASH DIET AND WEIGHT LOSS 135

CHAPTER 2: THE DASH DIET: HOW IT WORKS 137

TYPES OF DASH DIETS 137
TWO PHASES OF THE DASH DIET 138
DASH DIET: PHASE 1 139
DASH DIET: PHASE 2 140
A FEW TIPS BEFORE WE BEGIN 141
FIRST STEP: 141
MAKE A DETAILED MEAL PLAN AND GROCERY LIST: 142
PREPARE YOUR INGREDIENTS: 142
BASIC MISTAKES TO AVOID 142
EXCESSIVE CALORIE DEFICIT: 142
AVOIDING FATS: 143
LACKING VARIETY: 143

CHAPTER 3: KNOW YOUR CALORIES 144

ESTIMATES OF CALORIES BURNED DURING EXERCISE: 145

CHAPTER 4: GETTING STARTED: SETTING YOURSELF UP FOR SUCCESS 148

BRIEF OVERVIEW: 150
WHAT TO EAT DURING PHASE 1: 150
WHAT TO EAT DURING PHASE 2: 150
WHAT NOT TO EAT: 151
KNOW YOUR SERVING SIZES 151
PHASE 1 FOODS AND SERVINGS SIZES 151
PHASE 2 FOODS SERVINGS SIZES BY DAILY CALORIE COUNT 151

CHAPTER 5: GROCERY LIST 153

VEGETABLES: 154
WHOLE GRAINS: 155
FRUITS: 155
LEAN MEATS, POULTRY, AND FISH: 155
DAIRY PRODUCTS: 157
FATS AND OILS: 157
NUTS, SEEDS, AND LEGUMES: 158

SWEETS: 158
ALCOHOL: 159

CHAPTER 6: DASH DIET: THE ESSENTIALS 159

CHAPTER 7: LET'S GET STARTED STEP-BY-STEP 165

PART 1: STARTING THE DASH DIET 165
PART 2: START YOUR TWO-WEEK, PHASE 1 PROGRAM. 165
PART 3: TRANSITION TO PHASE 2, YOUR LIFELONG DASH DIET 166

CHAPTER 8: PHASE 1 MEAL PLAN 167

CHAPTER 9: DASH DIET RECIPES 170

BREAKFAST RECIPES 170
RECIPE 1: BREAKFAST SCRAMBLE 170
RECIPE 2: POACHED EGGS WITH AVOCADO AND TOMATO 171
RECIPE 3: SPINACH AND FETA OMELET 172
RECIPE 4: MUSHROOM AND ONION QUICHES 173
RECIPE 5: SHAKSHUKA (MIDDLE EASTERN EGGS AND TOMATO) 175

LUNCH RECIPES 177

RECIPE 6: CHICKEN SALAD SALAD 177
RECIPE 8: COLLARD GREEN LEAF CHICKEN WRAP 179
RECIPE 9: TUNA SALAD 180
RECIPE 10: GRILLED CHICKEN AND PINE NUT SALAD 181
RECIPE 11: ITALIAN EGGPLANT AND TOMATO 182

DINNER RECIPES 183

RECIPE 12: WALNUT CRUSTED SALMON 183
RECIPE 12: SESAME-MAPLE ROASTED TOFU 184
RECIPE 13: ROMAINE LEAF FISH TACO 186
RECIPE 14: CRISPY TOFU BLEND 187

RECIPE 15: VEG-KEBABS 189

Part 1

Introduction

The DASH diet, or Dietary Approaches to Stop Hypertension, has been called the best diet overall for 8 consecutive years by U.S. News and World Report. Here, I explore some history of the diet and the significant characteristics which led to its popularity.

The DASH diet was introduced in the 1990s when the National Institute of Health (NIH) started funding dietary intervention projects to help aiding medical conditions. The most significant characteristic of the diet is its proven health benefit to reduce high blood pressure. Hence the name, Dietary Approaches to Stop Hypertension.

The diet was created after researches noted an interesting correlation between the blood pressures of vegans or vegetarians and the general American public eating "American food". It was found that the blood pressure in vegans or vegetarians was markedly lower.
One of the main reasons the DASH diet helps people with hypertension is that it reduces salt consumption. It prescribes a lower sodium intake and includes calcium, potassium and magnesium — all of which help to lower blood pressure. There are two variants of the diet: Standard DASH diet which prescribes 1,500 mg of sodium and Low Sodium DASH diet which prescribes 1,500 mg of sodium.

Foods You Can Eat

The DASH diet allows one to eat a wide range of foods including:

- beans
- fruits
- vegetables
- low fat milk
- whole grains
- fish
- nuts
- poultry

Foods You Should Consume Moderately

The foods you must avoid, or eat in very moderate quantities, include:

- red meat (you can have a little)
- beverages with added sugars (you should try to avoid these)
- sweets (you can have a little)
- fats (you can have a little)

Health Benefits of the DASH Diet

The biggest health benefit of the DASH diet is that it helps to reduce high blood pressure. Furthermore, it's backed by major health organizations. For instance, the

DASH diet is recommended by American Heart Association and the National Heart, Lung, and Blood Institute.

A study by a team of researchers at Wake Forest School of Medicine in Winston Salem, North Carolina, found that the DASH diet reduced the risk of heart failure by a surprising half in people under the age of 75.

Another study has found that the diet may help in lowering depression. Some researchers have found an interesting correlation between vegetarians or vegans and depression: vegetarians or vegans are likely to have lower, or no depression as compared with the rest of the American population.

In other benefits, the diet helps to prevent osteoporosis, heart disease, cancer, diabetes and stroke.

Cons of the DASH Diet

I feel a need to list some cons of the diet, which are as follows:
- it's high maintenance
- it can get expensive
- there's no proper support system in place
- there's quite a bit of food tracking involved

BREAKFAST

Banana and Peanut Butter Smoothie

Ingredients
- One cup of milk, nonfat
- One tablespoon of natural peanut butter
- One medium fresh banana

Instructions
1. Place all the ingredients in your blender or food processor.
2. Blend until creamy smooth
3. Add ice if you desire the smoothie to be cooler
Serve immediately and enjoy.

Blueberry and Banana Breakfast Muffins

Serving: one muffin
180 Calories – Fat 5 gr. – Saturated Fat 4 gr. – Sodium 160 milligrams – Carbohydrates 31 gr. – Fiber 2 gr. – Sugar 12 gr. Protein 4 gr.

Ingredients

- ¾ cup of a ripe banana, masse
- ¾ cup + two tablespoons of almond milk, unsweetened
- ¼ cup of maple syrup
- 1 teaspoon of apple cider vinegar
- ¼ cup of melted coconut oil
- 6 tablespoons of cane sugar
- 1 teaspoon of vanilla extract
- 2 cups of white spelt flour
- 2 teaspoons of baking powder
- 1.5 teaspoons of ground cinnamon
- ½ teaspoon of baking soda
- ½ teaspoon salt
- ½ cup of chopped walnuts
- 1.25 cups of fresh or frozen blueberries

Instructions

1. Preheat your oven to 350° F.
2. Grease a muffin tin or place cupcake liners.
3. In a bowl, mash the ripe banana.
4. Place ¾ cup of mashed banana into another bowl with the almond milk, vinegar, vanilla extract and maple syrup. Set aside.

5. In a pot melt the coconut oil over low heat and set aside.
6. In another bowl combine the flour, baking powder, baking soda, sugar, cinnamon and salt.
7. Stir the coconut oil into the mashed banana mixture. Now pour the wet ingredients into the dry ingredients and combine gently.
8. Fold in the walnuts and blueberries. Do not over mix, blend gently.
9. Spoon in a ¼ cup of your batter into each muffin tin or cupcake liner. Place a couple of blueberries on top of each batter portion.
10. Bake for 25 minutes at 350° F. Cool for a t least 20 minutes before serving.

A Breakfast Casserole

Servings: Six

Ingredients

- 6 whisked large eggs
- 2/3 cup of milk
- 1 cup of cheddar cheese, shredded
- ½ teaspoon of salt
- 5 slices of whole wheat bread, one day old and cubed
- 4 strips of bacon which has been cooked and crumbled into bits
- 1 cup of cooked vegetables (onions, bell peppers and/or broccoli)

Instructions

1. Preheat your oven to 350° F.
2. Whisk the eggs in a bowl and then add in the cheese, milk and salt until the mixture is completely blended.
3. Soak the bread cubes in the egg mixture and blend gently.
4. Add in the crumbled bacon and cooked vegetables.
5. Now pour the mixture into a greased baking dish (8x8 inches) and bake for 45 minutes. The top should appear golden brown.
6. Serve warm.

Enjoy!

Cheddar, Kale and Pepper Frittata

Servings: Six to eight
Calories 77

Ingredients

- 12 eggs
- ¾ cup of milk
- 1 cup of cheddar cheese, shredded
- 1 diced red pepper
- 5 ounces of baby kale
- 1/3 cup of scallions, sliced
- 1 teaspoon of extra virgin olive oil + oil for greasing
- ¼ teaspoon of salt
- ¼ teaspoon of pepper

Instructions

1. Preheat your oven to 375° F.
2. Grease an 8.5 x 12 inch casserole dish with olive oil.
3. Heat the olive oil in a skillet. Add in the diced red pepper and sauté until tender, then add in the kale and continue sautéing for about three minutes.
4. Remove the peppers and kale to the casserole dish and arrange them evenly. Add in the sliced scallion pieces.
5. Beat the eggs together with the milk, salt, and pepper. Now pour the egg mixture into the pan over the vegetables. Sprinkle the cheese on the top of the egg and vegetable mixture.

6. Bake for about 40 minutes. The mixture should be slightly browned. Serve warm.
Enjoy!

Chocolate Smoothie

Servings: two 12-ounce servings
252 Calories – Fat 12 gr. – Saturated Fat 2 gr. – Carbohydrates 33 gr. – Fiber 8 gr. – Sugar 8 gr. – Protein 11 gr.

Ingredients

- 2 cups of vanilla soymilk
- ½ of a pitted and peeled avocado
- ¼ of a cup of cocoa powder, unsweetened
- 1 peeled medium banana
- 2 individual packets of sweetener

Instructions

1. Place all your ingredients into your blender or food processor. Combine until creamy smooth. Serve immediately.

French Cinnamon Toast

Servings: two servings of 2 slices each
299 Calories – Fat trace – Saturated fat trace – Sodium 334 mg. – Carbohydrates 57 gr. – Fiber <1 gr. – Protein 11 gr. – Sugar 17 gr.

Ingredients

- 4 egg whites
- 4 slices of cinnamon bread
- 1 teaspoon of vanilla extract
- ¼ cup of maple syrup
- ¼ teaspoon of cinnamon, ground
- 1/8 teaspoon of nutmeg, ground
- 2 teaspoons of powdered sugar

Instructions

1. Combine the egg whites together with the vanilla extract and ground nutmeg. Whisk until completely blended.
2. Dip the bread slices into the egg mixture making sure to coat both sides.
3. Place a nonstick skillet over medium heat. When the pan is sufficiently heated, add in the bread and sprinkle with ground cinnamon. Cook for about four minutes on each side until the bread is golden brown.
4. Place two slices of the French toast on individual plates. Add on 1 teaspoon of powdered sugar and 2 tablespoons of maple syrup to each portion. Serve immediately.

Cottage Cheese Pancakes

Servings: Four
511 Calories

Ingredients

- 1 cup of oat flour
- ½ cup of sorghum flour
- 2 tablespoons of teff flour
- 1 tablespoon of baking powder
- 1/3 cup plus one tablespoon of tapioca starch
- ½ teaspoon of salt
- ½ teaspoon of flax meal
- 3.5 teaspoons of sugar
- ¾ cup of buttermilk
- 3 eggs
- 1/3 cup of cottage cheese
- ½ teaspoon of vanilla extract
- ½ cup of maple syrup
- 1 pint of blueberries
- 4 teaspoons of canola oil
- 3 tablespoons of water
- 1 teaspoon of lemon juice

Instructions

1. Mix the flours, baking powder, starch, flax meal, salt and sugar in a bowl and combine evenly.
2. Whisk the buttermilk, eggs, cottage cheese, vanilla, and oil together in another bowl.
3. Create a well in the middle of your dry ingredients and begin to pour the wet ingredients in

the well slowly. Whisk and make sure that no lumps form.

4. Continue adding all the wet ingredients until you achieve a smooth batter. Set aside the batter for 15 minutes and preheat your skillet or griddle.

5. In the meantime, blend the blueberries, water, maple syrup, lemon juice and a pinch of salt into a pot and blend evenly. Heat over medium heat until blueberries pop. Set aside but keep warm.

6. Oil the preheated griddle with non-stick spray and spoon the batter onto the griddle.

7. Cook the pancakes about two minutes and flip to cook the other side.

8. Serve warm immediately with the blueberry-maple compote. Enjoy.

Granola Bars

Servings: Eighteen

Ingredients
- 2.5 cups of toasted rice cereal
- 2 cups of oatmeal
- ½ cups of raisins
- ½ cup of light corn syrup
- ½ cup of peanut butter
- ½ cup of brown sugar, firmly packed
- 1 teaspoon of vanilla extract

Instructions

1. Mix the rice cereal, raisins and oatmeal in a bowl and stir with a wooden spoon.
2. Mix the brown sugar and corn syrup in a saucepan and heat over medium high. Stirring constantly, bring the mixture to a boil. Once it boils, remove from heat.
3. Mix the peanut butter and vanilla extract into the sugar mixture. Stir until smooth.
4. Pour the peanut butter mixture into the bowl with the raisin mixture. Combine thoroughly.
5. Transfer the mixture and press into a 9x13 inch baking dish. Allow to cool completely and cut into bars. Enjoy with yogurt if so desired.

Oatmeal Breakfast in a Jar

Servings: one
518 Calories –

Ingredients

- ¼ cup of oatmeal
- ¾ cup of kefir
- 2 tablespoons of raisins
- 1 tablespoon of chia seeds
- 1 tablespoon of coconut flakes, unsweetened

Instructions

1. Place the ingredients inside a 16-ounce mason jar.
2. Close the lid securely and refrigerate overnight.
3. Remove the jar from the refrigerator, stir and enjoy.

Pineapple Smoothie

Servings: two
461 calories –

Ingredients

- ¾ cup of milk
- ½ cup of ice
- ¾ cup of pineapple chunks
- ¾ cup rinsed and drained canned chickpeas
- 2 teaspoons of turmeric, ground
- 2 tablespoons of almond butter
- 2 dates, pitted

Instructions

1. Combine all the ingredients in your blender or food processor. Blend until creamy smooth and enjoy.

Walnut and Honey Oats in a Jar

Servings: one

345 Calories – Fat 13 gr. – Saturated Fat 2 gr. – Sodium 53 mg. – Carbohydrates 53 gr. – Fiber 5 gr. – Sugar 31 gr. – Protein 10 gr.

Ingredients

- 1/3 cup of oats
- 1 tablespoon of honey
- 3 tablespoons of milk, fat-free
- ½ cup of assorted fresh fruit
- 3 tablespoons of plain yogurt, reduced fat
- 2 tablespoons of chopped toasted* walnuts

Instructions

1. Mix the oats, yogurt, milk, and honey in a mason jar. Place your fruit and walnuts on top of the mixture and seal. Refrigerate overnight.

To toast the walnuts, bake them in a pan for 5 to 10 minutes at 350°F, or brown them over low heat in a skillet.

Scrambled Eggs with Spinach and Mushrooms

Servings: one

Ingredients

- ½ cup of sliced fresh mushrooms
- 1 whole egg
- 2 egg whites
- 1 cup of fresh chopped spinach
- 2 tablespoons of feta cheese
- Pepper as desired
- Cooking spray

Instructions

1. Heat an 8-inch non-stick frying pan over a medium heat setting. Spray with cooking spray.
2. Add in the mushrooms and spinach and sauté them for three minutes. The spinach should wilt.
3. Whisk together the egg and egg whites in a bowl and add in the feta cheese and pepper and mix.
4. Pour the egg mixture over the mushrooms and spinach in the pan.
5. Cook the eggs for another 4 minutes while stirring with a spatula. The eggs should be completely cooked.

Sweet Potato Waffles with Honey and Blueberry Syrup

Servings: One waffle with ¼ cup of syrup
222 Calories – Fat 6 gr. – Saturated Fat 1 gr. – Carbohydrates 37 gr. – Fiber 3 gr. – Sodium 192 mg. – Sugar 14 gr. – Protein 5 gr.

Ingredients

For the waffles
- 1/3 cup of sweet potato, peeled and diced
- ¾ cup of all-purpose flour
- ¼ cup of cornmeal
- ¼ cup of whole-wheat flour
- 1 tablespoon of baking powder
- 1 egg white
- 1 cup of soymilk
- 1/8 teaspoon of cinnamon, ground
- ½ teaspoon of salt
- 1/8 teaspoon of ginger, ground
- 2 tablespoons light molasses
- 2 tablespoons of extra virgin olive oil

For the syrup
- 1.5 cups of blueberries
- 1 tablespoon of fresh lemon juice
- 1 teaspoon lemon zest, grated
- 1 tablespoon honey
- 1 tablespoon light molasses
- 2 tablespoons water
- pinch of cloves, ground

Instructions

1. To make the syrup mix the blueberries, water, honey, lemon zest and juice, molasses and pinch of cloves in a saucepan. Bring to a boil over medium heat. Once the mixture boils, reduce the heat to a low setting and cover and simmer for five minutes or until slightly thickened. Place aside and keep warm.

2. Prepare a saucepan half filled with water and bring to a boil. During this time peel and dice the sweet potato. Once the water boils, add in the diced sweet potato and bring to a boil again. Reduce the heat and simmer until the sweet potato becomes very tender. Drain and place in a blender and puree until creamy smooth. Set aside.

3. In a bowl, sift together the baking powder, cornmeal, flours, ginger, cinnamon, and salt. In another bowl, combine the potato puree, soymilk, molasses and olive oil. Now add in the flour mixture and stir to blend.

4. Beat the egg white with an electric mixture until peaks form. Now whisk in 1/3 of the egg white into the potato batter. Fold the remaining egg white into the batter until blended.

5. Heat the oven to 225° F and place a baking sheet inside. Heat the waffle iron. Spoon ½ cup of batter into the waffle iron and cook.

6. Transfer the waffle to a baking sheet to keep warm. When ready to serve, accompany with the blueberry honey syrup.

Vegetable Muffins

Servings: twelve

Ingredients

- 1 cup of chopped onion
- ¾ cup of shredded low-fat cheddar cheese
- 1 cup of chopped broccoli
- 4 eggs
- 1 cup of diced tomatoes
- 2 cups of non-fat milk
- 1 cup of baking mix for pancakes or biscuits
- ½ teaspoon of salt
- ½ teaspoon of pepper
- 1 teaspoon of Italian seasoning or dried basil and oregano

Instructions

1. Preheat your oven to 375° F. Oil twelve muffin tins or place in cupcake liners.
2. Place broccoli, onions, tomatoes and cheese into the muffin cups
3. In a bowl, beat the eggs, milk, baking mix, salt, pepper and seasoning until creamy smooth.
4. Pour the egg mixture over the ingredients already in the muffin liners
5. Bake for approximately 40 minutes until golden brown. Cool for five minutes. Serve and enjoy.

Lunch

Baked Zucchini & Cheese

Servings: two

Ingredients
- 1 medium-sized zucchini
- 1 teaspoon of extra-virgin olive oil
- 1/8 teaspoon of onion powder
- 1/8 teaspoon of garlic powder
- 2 tablespoons of Parmesan cheese, grated

Instructions

1. Preheat your oven to 375°F. Wash the zucchini and trim off the ends. At approximately every half inch in length, cut through the zucchini but not all the way. The zucchini slices should remain connected along the bottom.
2. Dry your zucchini with some paper towel and transfer it onto a piece of aluminum foil that can be completely wrapped around the zucchini.
3. Drizzle the zucchini with olive oil then sprinkle it with both the onion and garlic powders. Wrap the zucchini entirely in the foil, closing it and place on a baking sheet.
4. Bake the zucchini for about 35 minutes until tender. Remove from your oven and open the foil wrapping. Now sprinkle your zucchini with the Parmesan cheese. Leaving the foil open, return the

zucchini to the oven and bake for another two minutes. Serve while warm.

Guacamole Bean Cakes

Servings: four

Ingredients

- One 15 ounce can of black beans with low sodium
- One 7 ounce can of chipotle peppers in adobo sauce
- 2 garlic cloves
- 3 tablespoons of fresh cilantro
- 1 teaspoon of cumin, ground
- 2 slices of whole wheat bread
- 1 large egg
- ½ avocado
- 1 tablespoon of lime juice
- 1 plum tomato

Instructions

1. Tear up the two slices of bread into pieces and place in a food processor or blender. Blend until the bread is reduced to crumbs. Place the crumbs in a bowl and set aside for later.
2. Blend the cilantro and garlic together until chopped finely.
3. Drain and rinse the black beans and add to the cilantro garlic mixture. Add in one chipotle pepper and 2 teaspoons of the adobo sauce. Now blend together until the beans appear to be chopped coarsely.

4. Add this mixture to the breadcrumbs in the bowl and then add in the egg. Combine all the ingredients together well.
5. Form four patties. Grill your patties on a greased grill for 10 minutes until the patties have been heated through. Flip your patties once.
6. Mash the avocado in a bowl and add the lime juice, stirring. Use a pinch of salt and pepper to season.
7. Dice the tomato.
8. Serve the patties with the guacamole and diced tomato.

Beef Sautéed with Asparagus

Servings: four

Ingredients

- One pound of very lean beef sirloin or tenderloin without fat that has been sliced into very thin pieces
- 12 ounces of asparagus
- 1 peeled carrot, shredded
- 2 teaspoons of extra-virgin olive oil
- Freshly ground pepper
- Salt
- 1 teaspoon of dried crushed Provence herbs
- ½ cup of Marsala
- ¼ teaspoon of lemon peel, grated
- Hot boiled rice

Instructions

1. Clean, rinse and drain the asparagus, removing the fibrous ends. Cut the asparagus into two-inch pieces.
2. In a non-stick skillet over medium heat, warm the olive oil. When heated add in the beef and carrot together with salt and pepper, stirring for three to four minutes.
3. Add in the asparagus pieces and the Provence herbs. Cook for another three minutes.
4. Now add in the Marsala and lemon peel. Reduce the heat setting.
5. Cook for five minutes uncovered until the beef is done and the asparagus is tender but still crisp.

6. Serve over hot rice.

Chicken Burritos

Servings: four

For one burrito: Calories 286 - Fat 6 gr. – Saturated Fat 1 gr. - Carbohydrates 38 gr. - Fiber 9 gr. – Sodium 382 mg. – Sugar 9 gr. – Protein 20 gr.

Ingredients
- 4 whole wheat tortillas
- 1 teaspoon of extra-virgin olive oil
- 1 chopped red bell pepper
- 1 seeded and chopped jalapeno pepper
- 1 chopped onion
- 2 chopped ribs of celery
- 2 cups of grape tomatoes
- 2 tablespoons of cumin seeds
- 2 tablespoons of fresh oregano
- 2 chopped garlic cloves
- ½ cup of rinsed and drained canned black beans (no salt added)
- 2 cups of green cabbage, shredded
- 8 ounces of chicken breast meat, cooked

Instructions

1. Heat the oil in a large skillet over medium to high heat. Sauté the celery, cumin, onions, and peppers for 12 to 15 minutes until slightly browned.

2. Add in the garlic, oregano and tomatoes. Continue sautéing for another 8 to 10 minutes until the tomatoes are blistered and opened.
3. Transfer the mixture to your blender or food processor and blend to your preferred consistency.
4. Shred the cooked chicken breast meat and divide evenly in the four tortillas. Add in the cabbage, beans and your sauce. Roll and serve.

Chicken Noodle Soup

Servings: four

Ingredients

- 1 cup of cooked non-brined chicken cut into bite-sized pieces which has both skin and bones removed
- 1 teaspoon of extra-virgin olive oil
- 3 minced garlic cloves
- 1 cup of chopped onion
- 1 cup of chopped celery
- 1 cup of carrots, peeled and sliced
- 4 ounces of dried linguini noodles broken into pieces
- 2 tablespoons of chopped fresh parsley
- 4 cups of reduced sodium chicken broth

Instructions

1. In a large-sized saucepan heat the olive oil over medium heat. Sauté the onion and garlic until tender and translucent.
2. Add in the celery and the carrots and continue sautéing for another four minutes. Add in the chicken broth. Bring the mixture to a boil. Lower the heat, cover and simmer for five minutes.
3. Add in the linguini and stir the mixture until it boils again. Lower the heat, cover and simmer for ten to fifteen minutes making sure the pasta and vegetables are tender.
4. Add in the cooked chicken and fresh parsley. Heat and serve.

Greek Salad

Servings: eight
Serving size three cups
Calories 97 - Fat 5 gr. – Saturated Fat 1 gr. – Carbohydrates 10 gr.- Fiber 4 gr. – Sodium 158 mg. – Sugar 4 gr. – Protein 3 gr.

Ingredients

For the salad
- 1 unpeeled, seeded, and diced English cucumber
- 1 large 1.5 lbs. eggplant, cleaned, trimmed and cubed
- 1 seeded and diced tomato
- 1 lb. of steamed spinach, torn or cut into bite-sized pieces
- ½ diced red onion
- 2 tablespoons of chopped and pitted Greek black olives
- 2 tablespoons of feta cheese, crumbled
- Olive oil cooking spray

For the dressing
- 2.5 tablespoons of extra-virgin olive oil
- 1 tablespoon of red wine vinegar
- 2 teaspoons of chopped fresh oregano
- 1 tablespoon of fresh lemon juice
- ¼ teaspoon of salt
- ¼ teaspoon of freshly ground black pepper

Instructions

1. Heat the oven to 450° F.
2. To make the dressing whisk the lemon juice, vinegar, oregano, salt and pepper together in a bowl. During whisking, add in the olive oil slowly until blended and set aside.
3. Coat a baking sheet with olive oil cooking spray and place the eggplant cubes in a single layer. Spray the eggplant with the same oil cooking spray. Roast for ten to twelve minutes. Turn over the cubes and continue roasting until soft and golden. Set aside and allow to cool.
4. In a large salad bowl combine the cooled eggplant, cucumber, onion, spinach and tomato.
5. Pour over the dressing and toss the ingredients gently to cover evenly with the vinaigrette and mix well. Divide the salad evenly on four plates and sprinkle with olives and feta cheese. Serve.

Lemon Cod with Capers

Servings: four
Serving size one fillet – Calories 168 – Fat 4 gr. – Saturated fat 2 gr. – Carbohydrates 2 gr. – Fiber trace – Sodium 203 mg. – Sugar 0gr. – Protein 31 gr.

Ingredients

- 4 fillets of cod approximately 6 ounces each
- 1 cup of hot water
- 2 lemons
- 1 tablespoon of softened butter
- 1 teaspoon of low sodium chicken flavored bouillon granules
- 1 tablespoon of flour
- 4 teaspoons of rinsed and drained capers

Instructions

1. Preheat your oven to 350° F.
2. Spray four separate pieces of aluminum foil with cooking spray
3. Place 1 cod fillet on each aluminum foil square.
4. Cut one lemon into four halves. Squeeze the juice of a lemon half over the four fillets. Slice the remaining half into four slices and place a slice on each fillet and seal the foil for each fillet.
5. Place the fillets in the oven and bake for approximately twenty minutes until the fish is opaque throughout.

6. While the fillets bake, remove the peel from the remaining lemon. Only cut away the peel. Slice the peel into slices that are ¼ inch wide. Set aside for later.

7. In a bowl combine the bouillon granules with the hot water. Stir until they dissolve. Place aside.

8. In another bowl mix the butter with the flour. Place in a saucepan and heat on a medium setting until the mixture melts. Add the bouillon to the butter and flour mixture and stir until it thickens. Now add the capers and remove from the heat source.

9. Pour the sauce over the fish and serve garnished with a lemon peel.

Goat Cheese and Pepper Frittata

Servings: six

Ingredients

- 8 eggs
- 1 cup of sliced red bell pepper
- ½ goat cheese, crumbled
- 1 bunch of trimmed and sliced scallions
- 2 tablespoons of freshly chopped oregano
- 2 tablespoons of extra-virgin olive oil
- ½ teaspoon of salt
- ¼ teaspoon of freshly ground black pepper

Instructions

1. Preheat the broiler in your oven.
2. Whisk together the eggs, pepper, oregano and salt in a bowl.
3. Heat the olive oil in a non-stick skillet over medium heat. Add in the scallions and bell pepper and sauté, stirring always until the scallions are wilted, about one minute.
4. Pour the egg mixture over the sautéed vegetables and cook in the skillet for approximately three minutes. You can lift the edges to allow the egg to flow underneath. Dot the frittata with the goat cheese and place the pan in the oven under the broiler for about three minutes until golden. Remove and let rest for three minutes. The frittata can be served either hot or cold.

Primavera Pasta

Servings: six

Ingredients

- 1 lb. of penne pasta
- 3 sliced garlic cloves
- 2 tablespoons of extra-virgin olive oil
- 3 peeled and sliced carrots
- 24 halved cherry tomatoes
- 1 sweet red pepper
- 1 bunch of asparagus about 1 lb.
- 1 sweet yellow pepper
- ¾ teaspoon of salt
- ¼ teaspoon of freshly ground black pepper
- 2 tablespoons of Parmesan cheese, grated
- 2/3 cup of half-and-half

Instructions

1. Clean the asparagus and snap off the ends. Cut into 1-inch pieces.
2. Halve the sweet peppers. Remove the seeds and slice them into pieces.
3. Salt a large pot of water and bring to a boil. Add the pasta and cook until "al dente" tender but still firm.
4. While the pasta is cooking, heat a skillet over medium high heat. Add in the olive oil, and garlic and sauté for two minutes.
5. Add in the carrots and sauté for another five minutes. Reduce the heat to medium. Add in the asparagus and cover. Cook for ten minutes until

tender. Uncover the skillet and add in the peppers and cook for another 5 minutes. Stir.

6. Add in the cherry tomatoes, half-and-half, salt and pepper. Also stir in a ¼ cup of the pasta water.

7. Drain the pasta and place in a large-sized bowl.

8. Pour the sauce over the pasta and sprinkle with the Parmesan. Now toss gently. Serve immediately.

Roast Chicken with Gravy

Servings: four

Ingredients

- 1 Free range chicken approximately 3.5 lbs.
- 1 roughly chopped onion
- 1 halved lemon
- 2 roughly chopped carrots
- 1 tablespoon flour
- 250 ml chicken broth
- fresh thyme, 1 bunch

Instructions

1. Preheat your oven to 375° F.
2. Place the vegetables in the bottom of a roasting pan, which is the correct size for your chicken.
3. Season the cavity of the chicken with salt and pepper. Place the lemon halves and the thyme in the cavity.
4. Place the chicken on top of the vegetables in the roaster. Rub the breast and legs generously with butter, then season with salt and pepper.
5. Place in the oven and roast for one hour and twenty minutes.
6. Remove from oven and allow to rest for 15 minutes. As you remove the chicken allow the any juices (from the cavity as well) to run into the roaster.
7. While the chicken rests, make the gravy. Place your roaster over a low flame. Add in the flour. Gradually add in the chicken broth. Stir constantly until

you achieve a thickened sauce. Simmer for several minutes and scrape any browned bits from the pan. Strain your gravy into a saucepan and continue simmering. Season to taste. Serve with the chicken.

Salmon Chowder

Servings: eight
Calories 166 – Fat 2.5 gr. – Saturated Fat 0.5 gr. – Carbohydrates 26 gr. - Fiber 2 gr. – Sodium 207 mg. – Sugar 0 gr. – Protein 11 gr.

Ingredients

- 6 ounces of canned or pouched pink salmon
- ½ cup of celery, chopped
- 1 minced clove of garlic
- 1 cup of frozen carrots and peas
- 2.5 cups of frozen country style hash browns with green pepper and onion
- One 15 oz. can of reduced sodium chicken broth
- 1 teaspoon of extra-virgin olive oil
- ½ teaspoon of dill
- ½ teaspoon of freshly ground black pepper
- One 12 oz. can of evaporated skim milk
- 1 can (14 ¾ oz.) no added salt, creamed corn

Instructions

1. In a good-sized saucepan, sauté the olive oil and celery for ten minutes over medium heat. Add the minced garlic and sauté for another minute.
2. Add in the chicken broth, carrots and peas, hash browns, dill and pepper and bring the mixture to a boil. Lower your heat and simmer for ten minutes. The vegetables should be tender but not overcooked.

3. Add in pieces of the pink salmon, and then stir in the evaporated milk. Finally add in the corn. Cook the chowder until completely heated and serve warm.

Sloppy Joe Sandwiches

Servings: six
Serving size: one sandwich
Calories 251 – Fat 9 gr. – Saturated Fat 3 gr. – Carbohydrates 28 gr. – Fiber 4 gr. – Sodium 203 mg. - Sugar 0 gr. – Protein 19 gr.

Ingredients
- 1 pound of 90% lean ground beef
- 1 large onion, chopped
- 1 large green bell pepper, chopped
- 1 ½ cans of reduced sodium tomato soup (10.75 oz. each)
- 6 whole-wheat hamburger buns

Instructions
1. Cook the beef for ten minutes in a non-stick skillet together with the onion and pepper until the vegetables are tender and the meat is browned. Drain the mixture and then return it to the skillet.
2. Add in the tomato sauce to the ground beef mixture and mix well. Simmer for another ten to twelve minutes.
3. Place two thirds of a cup of the mixture onto the hamburger buns and serve immediately while hot.

Tuna Fish Salad

Servings: two

Ingredients

- One 5 oz. can of tuna in water, drained (preferably with less than 200 mg. sodium per serving)
- ¼ cup of chopped green onions
- 2 cups of arugula salad
- 1 cup of cooked bowtie or shell pasta (2 oz. dry)
- 1 tablespoon of extra-virgin olive oil
- 1 tablespoon of red wine vinegar
- 1 tablespoon of freshly shaved Parmesan cheese
- Freshly ground black pepper

Instructions

1. Place the tuna in a bowl together with the arugula, cooked pasta, onion, olive oil and vinegar. Toss together gently.
2. Divide the salad onto two individual plates. Top with Parmesan shavings and season with pepper.
3. Serve immediately.

Vegetable & Pasta Soup

Servings: twelve
Serving size: ¾ of a cup

Ingredients

- One 32 oz. box of reduced sodium chicken broth
- 6 minced cloves of garlic
- 1 cup of chopped onion
- 1.5 cups of carrots, coarsely shredded
- 1 cup of celery, thinly sliced
- 2 teaspoons of extra-virgin olive oil
- 4 cups of water
- 1.5 cups of dry ditalini pasta
- 2 tablespoons of fresh parsley, chopped
- ¼ cup of Parmesan cheese shavings

Instructions

1. In a 6-quart Dutch oven, heat the olive oil over a medium heat setting. Add in the minced garlic and sauté for a half-minute. Add in the carrots, celery and onions and continue to sauté, stirring for seven to eight minutes until tender.
2. Add in the chicken broth and the water and bring the mixture to a boil.
3. Add in the uncooked pasta and cook for another eight minutes or until your pasta is tender.
4. Top the individual servings with Parmesan cheese shavings and freshly chopped parsley.
5. Serve immediately.

Dinner

Baked Chicken with Rice

Servings: six
Calories 313 – Fat 3 gr. – Saturated Fat 1 gr. – Carbohydrates 38 gr. – Fiber 2.5 gr. – Sodium 104 mg. - Sugar 2 gr. – Protein 23 gr.

Ingredients
- 1 lb. of chicken breast halves, boneless and skinless
- 1 ½ cups of pearl onions
- 1 ½ cups of celery. Chopped
- 2 cups of chicken broth, unsalted
- 1 teaspoon of fresh tarragon
- ¾ cup of uncooked wild rice
- ¾ cup of uncooked long grain white rice
- 1 ½ cups of white wine

Instructions
1. Heat your oven to 300° F.
2. Cut the chicken breast halves into small pieces about 1 inch each. In a non-stick skillet, pour in one cup of the broth and add in the celery, chicken, onions and the tarragon. Cook for about ten minutes over medium heat under all the ingredients are tender. Place aside.
3. In a baking dish, mix the rice, white wine and remaining cup of broth. Allow the rice to soak for at least thirty minutes.

4. Finally add the chicken and vegetables to the mixture in the baking dish. Cover the baking dish and bake for one hour. Check on your dish every so often and add some extra broth, if the chicken appears dry. Serve immediately.

Baked Asian Marinated Salmon

Servings: two
Serving size: one fillet of salmon
Calories 247 – Fat 7 gr. – Saturated Fat 1 gr. – Carbohydrates 19 gr. – Fiber 2 gr. – Sodium 192 mg. - Sugar 0 gr. – Protein 27 gr.

Ingredients

- 2 salmon fillets, 4 oz. each
- 2 minced garlic cloves
- ¼ teaspoon of ground ginger
- ½ cup of pineapple juice without sugar added
- 1 teaspoon of low sodium soy sauce
- ¼ teaspoon of sesame oil
- 1 cup of diced fruit pieces (mango, papaya, pineapple, etc.)
- Freshly ground black pepper

Instructions

1. Mix the garlic, ginger, pineapple juice and soy sauce in a bowl. Place the salmon fillets in a baking dish and pour the mixture over the fish. Place the dish in the refrigerator and chill for one hour. Turn the salmon during this time.
2. Heat your oven to 375° F. Spray two squares of aluminum foil with cooking spray. Place the marinated salmon fillets on the aluminum foil squares. Drizzle the salmon with 1/8 teaspoon of sesame oil each. Sprinkle on the pepper and place ½ cup of diced fruit on each

fillet. Close the aluminum around the salmon and seal the edges.

3. Bake the salmon about ten minutes on each side until the fish is opaque. Place the salmon on warmed plates and serve immediately.

Beef Brisket

Servings: eight
Serving size: three oz. of sauce and three oz. of meat
Calories 229 – Fat 9 gr. – Saturated Fat 3 gr. – Carbohydrates 6 gr. – Fiber 1 gr. – Sodium 184 mg. - Sugar 0 gr. – Protein 31 gr.

Ingredients

- 2.5 lbs. beef brisket, with fat trimmed away
- 1 tablespoon of extra-virgin olive oil
- 1.5 cups of onions, chopped
- 4 peeled garlic cloves, smashed
- Freshly ground pepper
- 1 teaspoon of dried thyme flakes
- ¼ cup of red wine vinegar
- One 14.5 oz. can of tomatoes with liquid, no salt added
- 1 cup of beef broth, low-sodium

Instructions

1. Heat your oven to 350° F.
2. Cut the brisket into eight equal portions.
3. In a pot, heat the olive oil over medium heat. Season the brisket with the pepper and cook the meat making sure to brown it on all sides. Place the cooked brisket on a plate.
4. Place the onions in the pot and cook until browned. Add in the garlic and thyme and cook for another minute or two.

5. Add in the can of tomatoes with the liquid, the vinegar and the beef broth. Bring the mixture to a boil. Now place the beef back in the pot and place in the oven. Cook for approximately 3.5 hours until the beef is tender and serve.

Beef Stroganoff

Servings: four
Serving size: 2.5 cups
Calories 273 – Fat 5 gr. – Saturated Fat 2 gr. – Carbohydrates 37 gr. – Fiber 2 gr. – Sodium 193 mg. - Sugar 0 gr. – Protein 20 gr.

Ingredients

- ½ lb. of boneless beef round steak with all fat removed, approximately ¾" cut
- ½ cup of onion, chopped
- ½ cup of cream of mushroom soup, fat-free, undiluted
- 1 tablespoon of flour
- ½ cup of water
- ½ teaspoon of paprika
- ½ cup of sour cream, fat-free
- 4 cups of uncooked, yolkless egg noodles

Instructions

1. Sauté the onions in a non-stick skillet over medium heat for approximately five minutes until translucent. Add in the beef and cook for five more minutes. The beef should be browned and tender. Drain and set aside.
2. Fill a large pot with water and bring to a boil. Add in the noodles and cook until they are "al dente"….tender but not overcooked for about ten to twelve minutes. Drain the pasta well.

3.   Whisk together the soup, flour and water in a saucepan over medium heat. The sauce should thicken after about five minutes of cooking. Add in the paprika and pour over the beef in the skillet. Stir the mixture well until thoroughly warmed. Remove from the heat source and add in the sour cream. Mix well.

4.   Divide the pasta while still warm onto two plates and top with the beef mixture. Serve immediately.

Curried Pork Tenderloin

Servings: six
Serving size about 3 ounces
Calories 244 – Fat 8 gr. – Saturated Fat 2 gr. – Carbohydrates 19 gr. – Fiber 2 gr. – Sodium 48 mg. - Sugar 13 mg. – Protein 24 gr.

Ingredients

- 16 ounces of pork tenderloin
- 1 tablespoon of extra-virgin olive oil
- 1.5 tablespoons of curry powder
- 2 medium onions, chopped
- 1 tart apple, peeled and seeded
- 2 cups of apple cider, divided
- 1 tablespoon of corn starch

Instructions

1. Cut the pork tenderloin into six equal pieces. Chop the apple into chunks.
2. Season the pork pieces with the curry and set aside for 15 minutes.
3. Heat the olive oil in a skillet over medium heat. Add in the pork pieces and brown on both sides for about five minutes per side. Remove the pork and set aside.
4. Add in the onions to the skillet and sauté until tender and golden. Add in 1.5 cups of the apple cider, reduce the heat setting and simmer until the liquid has been reduced by half.

5. Add in the apple pieces, the remaining apple cider and the cornstarch. Simmer for about two minutes until the sauce thickens. Return the pork pieces to the skillet and simmer for five more minutes.
6. Place the pork loin on plates and pour the sauce over the meat. Serve immediately.

Spicy Pork Medallions

Servings: four
Serving size two medallions
Calories 219 – Fat 11 gr. – Saturated Fat 2 gr. – Carbohydrates 5 gr. – Fiber 1 gr. – Sodium 392 mg. - Sugar 2 gr. – Protein 25 gr.

Ingredients
- 1 lb. pork tenderloin, trimmed of fat
- 1 tablespoon of minced green onion
- 3 minced garlic cloves
- 1 tablespoon of extra-virgin olive oil
- 2 tablespoons of soy sauce, low-sodium
- ¾ teaspoon five-spice powder
- ¼ cup of dry white wine
- ½ cup of water with eventual extra tablespoons
- 1/3 cup of onion, chopped
- 1 tablespoon of chopped fresh parsley
- ½ head of cabbage, sliced thinly

Instructions
1. Prepare the marinade by combining the soy sauce, garlic, green onion, and spice powder in a baking dish. Whisk well. Add in the pork and turn over once making sure to coat the meat. Cover the baking dish and refrigerate overnight. Turn the pork occasionally.
2. Heat your oven to 400° F.
3. Remove the pork from the marinade and dry. Discard the marinade sauce. In an oven proof skillet, heat the olive oil over medium heat. Add in the pork

and cook for about five minutes browning on all sides. Add ½ cup of water to the skillet.

4. Place the pan in the oven and roast the pork until it is slightly pink inside. A thermometer inserted in the meat should read 160° F. Place the pork on a cutting board and cover with a clean towel. Allow the meat to rest for ten minutes.

5. Place the pan over medium heat and add in the wine. Scrape any brown bits from the pan with a wooden spoon. Add in the onion and cook for a minute. Add in the cabbage and an extra tablespoon of water. Reduce the heat a bit, cover and simmer until the cabbage wilts about five minutes. Add water if necessary.

6. Slice the pork into eight medallions. Divide the medallions and cabbage among four plates and garnish with parsley. Serve immediately.

Chicken with a Honey Crust

Servings: two
Serving size: one chicken breast
Calories 219 – Fat 3 gr. – Saturated Fat 1 gr. – Carbohydrates 21 gr. – Fiber 1 gr. – Sodium 187 mg. - Sugar 11 gr. – Protein 27 gr.

Ingredients

- 2 chicken breasts, 4 ounces each, boneless and skinless
- 1 teaspoon paprika
- 4 teaspoons of honey
- 8 saltine crackers (2 inch squares)

Instructions

1. Preheat the oven to 375°F. Spray a baking dish with cooking spray.
2. Crush the crackers in a bowl and add in the paprika. Mix well.
3. In another bowl, place the chicken with the honey. Toss the chicken in order to coat well. Add in the cracker and paprika mixture. Press the chicken into the cracker mix and coat evenly on both sides.
4. Place the chicken breasts in the baking dish and bake until cooked through and lightly browned for approximately 25 minutes. Serve immediately.

Lasagna

Servings: eight
Serving size: 1 slice (3 by 4 inches)
Calories 425 – Fat 13 gr. – Saturated Fat 6 gr. – Carbohydrates 42 gr. – Fiber 3.5 gr. – Sodium 500 mg. - Sugar 6 gr. – Protein 33 gr.

Ingredients

- 1 lb. ground beef, extra lean
- One 6 oz. can of tomato paste, unsalted
- One 8 oz. can of tomato sauce, unsalted
- 1 chopped onion
- ¾ teaspoon of garlic powder
- ¾ teaspoon of oregano
- 1.5 teaspoons of dried basil flakes
- 3.5 cups of water
- 1 cup of cottage cheese, low-fat
- 3 cups of shredded mozzarella cheese, low-fat
- ¾ lb. of uncooked lasagna noodles

Instructions

1. Heat your oven to 325° F. Coat a rectangular baking dish (9 x 13 inch) with cooking spray.
2. Prepare the sauce by combining the beef and onion in a saucepan. Cook over medium heat until the onion is translucent and the beef in browned. Drain the mixture well. Add in the basil, garlic powder, oregano, tomato paste, tomato sauce and water. Mix well and bring to a boil. Reduce the heat and simmer for 10 minutes.

3.   Place ½ cup of the sauce in the baking dish. Place a layer of uncooked lasagna noodles over the sauce. Place another 1/3 cup of sauce on the noodles followed by 1/3 cup of cottage cheese and one cup of mozzarella cheese. Repeat until you have used up all the ingredients.

4.   Cover the dish with aluminum foil and bake for approximately one hour and twenty minutes until the noodles are soft and the cheese is golden.

N.Y. Strip Steak with Whiskey Sauce

Servings: two
Serving size: one steak
Calories 330 – Fat 17 gr. – Saturated Fat 6 gr. – Carbohydrates 4 gr. – Fiber 1 gr. – Sodium 96 mg. - Sugar 2 gr. – Protein 24 gr.

Ingredients

- 2 New York strip steaks, 4 oz. each, trimmed of fat
- 3 chopped garlic cloves
- 2 oz. of button mushrooms
- 2 oz. of shiitake mushrooms, sliced
- 1 teaspoon of margarine, trans-free
- ¼ teaspoon of rosemary
- ¼ teaspoon of thyme
- ¼ cup of whiskey

Instructions

1. Coat a grill or broiler pan with cooking spray. Prepare a hot fire in a grill or prepare a broiler. The grill should be four to six inches from the heat source.
2. Grill or broil the steaks for about ten minutes on each side, until they are slightly pink on the inside. A food thermometer will indicate 145°F for medium rare, 160°F for medium or 170°F for well-done.
3. In a saucepan, over medium heat melt the margarine. Add in the garlic, mushrooms, rosemary and thyme. Sauté for two minutes until the mushrooms are tender. Remove from the heat source and add in

the whiskey. Stir for a minute. Top the steaks with the whiskey and mushroom sauce and serve.

Pasta with Tomatoes, Asparagus and Goat Cheese

Servings: due
Serving size: 2.5 cups
Calories 396 – Fat 8 gr. – Saturated Fat 4 gr. – Carbohydrates 64 gr. – Fiber 10 gr. – Sodium 142 mg. - Sugar 0 gr. – Protein 17 gr.

Ingredients

- 1/3 lb. of whole-wheat pasta (penne)
- ½ cup of cherry tomatoes
- ½ cup of asparagus, chopped into 1-inch pieces
- 1 tablespoon of water
- 1 tablespoon of minced garlic
- ¼ cup of fresh basil, chopped
- 2 oz. of goat cheese
- 1/8 teaspoon of freshly ground black pepper

Instructions

1. Fill a large pot with water and bring to a boil. Add in the pasta and cook for ten to twelve minutes until the penne are "al dente", tender but not over cooked. Drain thoroughly.
2. While the past cooks, place the asparagus pieces in a microwave bowl with the water. Heat on high for three minutes.
3. Combine the basil, cherry tomatoes, garlic and pepper in a bowl. Add in the asparagus and goat cheese, and eventually the pasta when cooked. Toss together well.

4. Refrigerate for twenty minutes to cool. Divide the pasta between two plates and serve. Garnish with a few fresh basil leaves if so desired.

Shepherd's Pie

Servings: six
Serving size: 1.5 cups
Calories 258 – Fat 7 gr. – Saturated Fat 3 gr. – Carbohydrates 19 gr. – Fiber 2 gr. – Sodium 413 mg. - Sugar 6 gr. – Protein 29 gr.

Ingredients

- 2 medium russet potatoes, cut into cubes
- ½ cup of chopped onions
- ½ cup of chopped carrots
- 1 teaspoon of extra-virgin olive oil
- 1 tablespoon of tomato paste
- 1 lb. of ground beef, lean
- ½ lb. of turkey breast, ground
- 1 teaspoon of fresh thyme, finely chopped
- 1 teaspoon of fresh rosemary, finely chopped
- ½ teaspoon of salt + ¼ teaspoon of salt
- ¼ teaspoon of freshly ground black pepper
- 2 cups of chicken broth
- ½ cup of thawed frozen peas
- ½ cup of thawed frozen corn
- 1 cup of skim milk
- 1 tablespoon of butter

Instructions

1. Heat your oven to 400° F. Place the potatoes in a pot with water and bring to a boil. Cook for about twenty minutes until soft.

2.   While the potatoes cook, heat the olive oil in a pan over medium heat. Add in the onions and carrots and sauté until tender. Now add in the beef and turkey. Beak the meat apart while sautéing. When the meat is thoroughly cooked, add in the pepper, rosemary, ½ teaspoon salt, thyme, and tomato paste. Add in the broth and simmer for ten minutes. Add in the peas and corn. Simmer the mixture until most of the broth has evaporated.

3.   Place the mixture in a baking or casserole dish.

4.   Once the potatoes are ready, drain the water and return the potatoes to the pot over a medium heat setting. Add in the butter, milk and ¼ teaspoon salt. Use a potato masher or electric hand mixer and mash the potatoes until smooth.

5.   Spread the potatoes over the meat mixture and bake for twenty minutes. Serve hot.

Shrimp Kebab

Servings: two
Serving size: one skewer
Calories 105 – Fat 1 gr. – Saturated Fat 0 gr. – Carbohydrates 0 gr. – Fiber 0 gr. – Sodium 185 mg. - Sugar 0 gr. – Protein 24 gr.

Ingredients
- 12 pieces of peeled and deveined shrimp
- 1 juiced lemon
- 2 teaspoons of finely mince garlic
- 1 tablespoon of extra-virgin olive oil
- 1 teaspoon of fresh tarragon, finely chopped
- 1 teaspoon of fresh rosemary, finely chopped
- ½ teaspoon of salt
- ¼ teaspoon of freshly ground pepper
- 2 wooden skewers at least 8 inches each

Instructions
1. Soak the skewers in water for ten to fifteen minutes.
2. Preheat a grill to high.
3. Mix the garlic, herbs, lemon juice, seasonings and olive oil together in a bowl.
4. Place the pieces of shrimp in the marinade sauce and set aside for ten minutes.
5. Skewer the marinated shrimp and grill for two minutes on each side or until the shrimp is completely cooked.

Roasted Lemons and Swordfish

Servings: four
Serving size: one fillet
Calories 280 – Fat 12 gr. – Saturated Fat 3 gr. – Carbohydrates 0 gr. – Fiber 0 gr. – Sodium 287 mg. - Sugar 4 gr. – Protein 34 gr.

Ingredients

- Four 6 oz. swordfish fillets
- 2 quartered lemons with seeds removed
- ½ teaspoon of chopped garlic
- ½ teaspoon of canola oil
- 1 tablespoon of sugar
- ¼ cup of fresh parsley, chopped
- ¼ teaspoon of salt

Instructions

1. Heat your oven to 375° F.
2. Place the lemon wedges in a bowl with the sugar and salt. Toss the wedges to cover evenly.
3. Place the wedges in a baking dish and cover the dish with aluminum foil. Roast for an hour until soft and browned.
4. Heat your broiler. Lightly coat a baking dish with cooking spray.
5. Place the fish into the baking dish and brush each with canola oil and sprinkle with garlic.
6. Broil the fish for five minutes on each side until opaque.

7. Place the fish on individual plates. Squeeze a roasted lemon wedge over each fillet and sprinkle with the fresh parsley. Serve with a lemon wedge.

Turkey and Broccoli Crepe

Servings: four
Serving size: one crepe
Calories 223 – Fat 7 gr. – Saturated Fat 4 gr. – Carbohydrates 23 gr. – Fiber 3 gr. – Sodium 200 mg. - Sugar 14 gr. – Protein 17 gr.

Ingredients
- 4 prepackage crepes
- 2 cups of broccoli, chopped
- ½ cup of reduced fat Colby jack cheese, finely shredded
- 4 oz. of sliced reduced sodium turkey breast

Instructions
1. Heat the oven to 350° F. Spray a banking dish with cooking spray.
2. Place a steamer basket in a pot and one inch of water and bring to a boil. Add in the broccoli and steam, covered, for seven minutes until crisp but tender.
3. Heat the crepes in your microwave for a minute or following the package indications.
4. Place ¼ of the turkey breast together with ¼ cup of the steamed broccoli and two tablespoons of cheese on each crepe. Roll the crepes up and place in the

baking dish with the seam-side underneath. Bake for five minutes until the cheese has melted. Serve immediately while hot.

Desserts

Apple Tart

Ingredients
Filling:
- ¼ cup of apple juice
- ½ cup of cranberries, dried
- 4 tart apples (large), cored, sliced and peeled
- ¼ tsp of ground cinnamon
- 1 tsp of vanilla extract
- 2 tsp of sugar
- 2 Tbsp of cornstarch

Crust:
- ¼ cup of ice water
- 1 ¼ cups of whole wheat flour
- 2 tsp of sugar
- 3 Tbsp of margarine (trans-free)

Instructions
1. ***For the filling:*** Preheat the oven to 375 F.
2. Mix the apple juice and cranberries in a small bowl that's safe for use in a microwave oven. Set the microwave to high and cook for 1 minute (cook for 30

seconds at a time and stir, until the juice is hot). Cover it and set it aside for about 1 hour.

3. Mix the apple slices and cornstarch in a large bowl. Toss them thoroughly so they're evenly coated. Pour into them the apple juice mixture and mix them well, stirring in the cinnamon and vanilla as well. Now set it aside.

4. **For the crust:** in a large sized mixing bowl, pour the flour and sugar. Cut the margarine and add it to the mixture until its crumbly. Mix 1 Tbsp of ice water at a time using a fork to make the dough.

5. On the countertop, tape a large piece of aluminum foil and drizzle it with some flour. Put the dough in the middle and flatten it. Now, roll the dough from the center to the edges using a rolling pin (we will try to make a circle with a diameter of about 13").

6. Spread the filling onto the dough, leaving a border area of 1-2". Now fold the edges on top of the filling. Sprinkle 2 tsp of sugar on it.

7. Remove the tape from the countertop and foil and place another piece of foil over the tart area (we do this to protect the fruit filling that's exposed).

8. Take a cookie sheet and slide in it the tart, including the foil and bake for about 30 minutes.

9. Remove the foil and bake it for about 10 more minutes, until it's brown.

10. Cut it into 8 slices and serve.

Enjoy.

Banana & Berry Ice cream

Ingredients
- One cup of frozen berries
- ½ cup of nonfat milk
- 1 ½ tsp of vanilla extract
- 3 bananas (frozen), large and cut into 1" pieces

Instructions

1. Place the peeled and sliced bananas in the freezer overnight (or for at least 8 hours).
2. Add the bananas, milk and vanilla in a food processor and process for about 1-2 minutes.
3. When the banana breaks down, stop the food processor and scrape its sides. Continue again until the mixture attains a soft consistency (while stopping, as needed, to scrape the sides of the bowl).
4. Add to the mixture the berries and pulses until they're thoroughly mixed.
5. Serve immediately.

Enjoy.

Tip: The base of this dessert is frozen bananas. You may substitute the bananas for cream which will remove the calories, cholesterol and fat from the dessert without interfering with flavor or creaminess.

Carrot Cake Cookies

Ingredients
- ½ cup of applesauce
- 1 ½ cup of carrots, finely grated
- 1 cup of flour
- ½ cup of light brown sugar (packed)
- ½ cup of oil
- 1 cup of raisins or golden raisins
- 2 cups of raw rolled oats (old-fashioned)
- ½ cup of sugar
- 1 cup of whole wheat flour
- Two eggs
- 1 tsp of baking powder
- 1 tsp of baking soda
- 1 tsp of ground cinnamon
- ½ tsp of ground ginger
- ½ tsp of ground nutmeg
- ¼ tsp of salt
- 1 tsp of vanilla

Instructions
1. Preheat the oven to 350 F.
2. Blend the applesauce, eggs, oil, sugars and vanilla.
3. Stir all the dry ingredients and mix them with the egg mixture. Stir it with the carrots and raisins.
4. Place the mixture on the cookie sheet using a teaspoon.

5. Bake in the preheated oven for about 12-15 minutes or until the mixture turns golden brown in color.
6. Store it in an airtight box.

You can also layer pudding with mixed berries or banana slices to make a healthy DASH dessert.

Carrot Raisin Tea Bread

Servings: eighteen

Nutrition per serving: Calories 144 – Fat 4 gr. – Sodium 140 mgr. – Carbs 25 gr. – Fiber 3 gr. – Sugar 14 gr. – Protein 2 gr.

Ingredients

- ½ cup of applesauce, unsweetened
- ½ cup of brown sugar
- 2 cups of carrots, shredded
- ¼ cup of honey
- ¼ cup of flaxseed flour
- ½ cup of olive oil
- 2/3 cups of raisins
- 1 ½ cup of whole wheat pastry flour
- ½ tsp of almond extract
- 1 ½ tsp of baking powder
- ½ tsp of baking soda
- ¼ tsp of cloves
- ¼ tsp of ground cayenne pepper
- ½ tsp of nutmeg
- ½ tsp of salt
- 1 Tbsp of cinnamon
- 1 Tbsp of lemon zest, grated
- Two eggs

Instructions

1. Heat the oven to 375 F.

2. In a large bowl, mix thoroughly the baking powder, baking soda, flaxseed flour, salt, spices and wheat flour.

3. Mix the almond extract, applesauce, eggs, honey, olive oil and sugar. Stir the mixture in carrots, lemon zest and raisins.

4. Blend the dry ingredients in the wet ingredients.

5. Lightly grease a 9x5" loaf pan and pour in it the batter. Bake in the preheated oven at 375 F for about 45-60 minutes.

6. Let it cool and cut into 1/2" slices.

Enjoy.

Chocolate Cake

Ingredients
- ½ cup of canola oil
- 1 cup of sugar
- 2 cups of water
- 3 cups of whole wheat pastry flour
- 3 Tbsp of cocoa powder, unsweetened
- 1 Tbsp of vanilla
- 2 Tbsp of vinegar
- 2 ¼ tsp of baking soda
- ½ tsp of salt

Instructions
1. Preheat the oven to 350 F.
2. In a 9x13" ungreased baking pan, put the baking soda, cocoa powder, flour, salt and sugar and stir them together using a whisk.
3. Make three holes in your dry mixture using a spoon. In the first hole, pour the oil. In the second, vanilla and in the third, vinegar.
4. Pour boiling water gently and evenly over the mixture in the pan, mixing everything with a whisk for about 2 minutes. Make sure there are no remains of dry ingredients in the mixture.
5. Bake the mixture for about 25-30 minutes. You can check if its baked properly by inserting a toothpick – it the toothpick comes out clean, you'll know its baked.
6. Let the cake cool fully.

7. Cut it into twenty squares and serve. Enjoy.

Fig Bars

Ingredients

- 16 oz of dried figs, chopped and stemmed
- 1 ½ cups of all-purpose flour
- 1 cup of brown sugar, packed
- ¼ cup of orange juice
- 1 ¼ cups of rolled oats (old-fashioned)
- ½ cup of softened margarine
- 1/3 cup of sugar
- ½ cup of walnuts, chopped
- 2 Tbsp of hot water
- One large egg
- ½ tsp of baking soda

Instructions

1. Preheat the oven to 350 F.
2. Either spray a 9x13" baking pan or oil it lightly.
3. In a mixing bowl, mix together the figs, orange juice, sugar, walnuts and hot water. Set the mixture aside.
4. Beat the margarine and brown sugar (they should give a creamy mixture). Mix it with the egg until it gives a smooth consistency.
5. Combine the baking soda and flour and stir into the egg mixture. Blend the oats with the mixture to prepare a soft dough. Set aside 1 cup of the dough for the purpose of topping.
6. Press your fingertips gently into the flour so that they're covered with it. Now press them onto the

remaining dough to make a thin layer of it at the bottom of the pan.
7.   Evenly spread the fig mixture on the dough surface and pat it. On the top, pour the crumbled dough that you set aside using a teaspoon.
8.   Bake for about 30 minutes or until they're golden brown in color. Allow them to cool down fully.
9.   Cut them in 1x3" bars.
Enjoy.

Fruitcake

Servings: twelve

Nutrition per serving: Calories 229 – Fat 5 gr. – Sodium 117 mgr. – Carbs 41 gr. – Fiber 5 gr. – Sugar 25 gr. – Protein 5 gr.

Ingredients

- ½ cup of apple juice, unsweetened
- ½ cup of applesauce, unsweetened
- 2 cups of dried fruit assorted and chopped. It can be cherries, currants, dates, figs, or their likes.
- ½ cup of drained, crushed pineapple (packed in juice)
- ¼ cup of flaxseed flour
- ½ cup of rolled oats
- ¼ cup of sugar
- ½ cup of walnuts, crushed or chopped
- 1 cup of whole wheat pastry flour
- Juice and zest of one lemon
- Juice and zest of one medium orange
- 2 Tbsp of real vanilla extract
- ½ tsp of baking powder
- ½ tsp of baking soda
- One egg

Instructions

1. Mix together the applesauce, dried fruit, fruit zests and juices, pineapple and vanilla in a medium bowl. Allow it to soak for about 15-20 minutes.
2. Line a 9x4" loaf pan with parchment paper.

3. Blend together the baking powder, baking soda, flours, oats and sugar in a large bowl. In this dry mixture, pour the fruit and liquid mixture and stir. Add to this the egg and walnuts and mix fully.

4. Pour the mixture in the pan and bake at 325 F for about 1 hour. To check if it's baked properly, insert a toothpick and see if it comes out clean.

5. Allow the cake to cool for about 30 minutes before removing.

Enjoy.

Milk Chocolate Pudding

Ingredients
- 2 Tbsp of cocoa powder
- 3 Tbsp of cornstarch
- 2 Tbsp of sugar
- 1/8 tsp of salt
- ½ tsp of vanilla
- 1/3 cup of chocolate chips
- 2 cups of nonfat milk

Instructions

1. Blend the cocoa powder, cornstarch, salt and sugar in a medium saucepan. Whisk the mixture in milk and heat over a medium flame while stirring until it thickens or begins to bubble.
2. Remove it from the flame and stir it with the chocolate chips and vanilla until the chips melt and pudding gives a smooth consistency.
   3. Either pour it in one large dish or four small dishes and chill them. *You might want to wrap the surface of the pudding with a plastic paper to prevent a skin from forming.*

Enjoy.

You may add sliced bananas or strawberries as toppings. And for a dose of omega-3 fatty acids, you may sprinkle ground flaxseed over the pudding.

Mint & Chocolate Brownies

Ingredients
- ½ cup of all-purpose flour
- ¼ cup of cocoa
- 2 cups of mini marshmallows
- 1 cup of sugar
- ½ teaspoon of salt
- 1 teaspoon of vanilla extract
- 4 ounces of butter
- 8 ounces of chocolate chips (semi-sweet)
- 3 eggs
- 25 peppermint patties (mini)

Instructions
1. Preheat the oven to 350 F.
2. Put the butter and chocolate in a stove and heat on a very low flame. Remove them from the heat and whisk in the eggs. Also, add cocoa, flour, salt and sugar to the mixture and mix thoroughly.
3. Take a 9x3" baking pan and line it with tin foil. Butter the entire foil and pour the brownie mixture in the pan. Place the patties on top and pour the remaining batter onto them.
4. Bake it for about 45 minutes and drizzle marshmallows on top. Now, broil for about 2-5 minutes until the marshmallows are light brown in color.
5. Allow it to cool for at least one hour. Cut it with a knife when it's cool (when you cut it, spray your knife with cooking spray or the marshmallows will stick to

the knife). If it's hard to cut, you can use scissors along with the knife.
Enjoy!

Oatmeal Chocolate Chip Cookies

Ingredients
- ½ cup of all-purpose flour
- 1 cup of chocolate chips, semisweet or bittersweet
- 2/3 cups of light brown sugar, packed
- 2/3 cups of sugar, granulated
- ½ cup of pastry flour (whole wheat)
- 2 cups of rolled oats
- ½ cup of tahini (Paste made from ground sesame seeds. It's available in natural food stores and some supermarkets)
- ½ cup of walnuts, chopped
- ½ tsp of baking soda
- 1 tsp of ground cinnamon
- ½ tsp of salt
- 4 Tbsp of cold butter (unsalted), cut into pieces
- 1 Tbsp of vanilla extract
- One large egg
- One large egg white

Instructions
1. Place the oven racks in the upper third and lower third of the oven and preheat to 350 F.
2. Take two baking sheets and line them with parchment paper.
3. In a medium sized bowl, whisk the baking soda, cinnamon, flour, whole wheat flour, oats and salt.

4. Blend the butter and tahini together – so that they form a paste – by beating them with an electric mixer. Add to it the brown sugar and granulated sugar and continue to beat the mixture. Now, pour in the egg, egg white and vanilla and beat them in. Stir with a wooden spoon until the mixture is moist. Then stir in the walnuts and chocolate chips.

5. Making sure your hands are damp, roll 1 Tbsp of the batter so it forms a ball. Place it on the baking sheet and flatten it but don't crack its sides. Repeat the same method with the remaining batter and place the bowls approximately 2" apart from each other.

6. Bake the cookies for about 16 minutes, or until they turn golden brown.

7. Allow the cookies to cool on the pans for about 2 minutes. Then place them in a wire rack to cool fully. Then bake another batch after the pans have cooled down.

8. You can store the cookies in an airtight container for about 2 days or freeze them if you need to store them for long.

Enjoy!

You can serve this with a tall glass of nonfat milk to make this the ultimate DASH combination of dairy and whole grains.

Parfait Americana

Servings: four

Nutrition per serving: Calories 129 – Fat 1 gr. – Sodium 144 mgr. – Carbs 24 gr. – Fiber 3 gr. – Sugar 1 gr. – Protein 6 gr.

Ingredients

- 1 ½ cup of blueberries (fresh)
- 1 pint of strawberries (fresh), sliced

For the Filling:

- 1/4 cup of cream cheese (fat-free), softened
- 1 cup of low-fat vanilla yogurt (artificially sweetened)
- 1 tsp of honey

Instructions

1. For the filling, beat the cream cheese, honey and yogurt in a bowl until they're fluffy.
2. Take parfait glasses and place 1/3 cup of strawberries in each. On top, put 3 Tbsp of the creamy filling and ¼ cup of blueberries. Garnish each with the remaining topping.
3. Serve it chilled.

Enjoy!

Peach Crumble

Ingredients

- Juice of one lemon
- 8 peaches (ripe), peeled, pitted and sliced
- 1/3 tsp ground cinnamon
- ¼ tsp of ground nutmeg
- 2 Tbsp of margarine (trans-free), cut into thin slices
- ¼ cup of dark brown sugar, packed
- ¼ cup of quick cooking oats
- ½ cup of whole wheat flour

Instructions

1. Preheat the oven to 375 F.
2. Spray a 9" pie-pan with nonstick cooking spray.
3. Place the peach slices in the pan and sprinkle cinnamon, lemon juice and nutmeg on top.
4. Whisk the flour and brown sugar in a small bowl. Then, using your fingers, crumble the margarine into the mixture. Now add the oats and keep stirring until it's evenly mixed. Sprinkle the mixture on top of the peaches.
5. Place the peaches in the oven and bake for about 30 minutes, or until they're soft and the topping turns brown. Cut into eight slices and serve warm.

Enjoy!

Pumpkin Pie

Ingredients
- ½ cup of egg whites
- 1 cup of ginger snaps
- ½ cup of sugar
- 16 oz. of pumpkin, canned
- 12 oz. can of evaporated skim milk
- 2 tsp of pumpkin pie spice

Instructions
1. Preheat the oven to 350 F.
2. Spray a 9-inch glass pie pan lightly with cooking spray.
3. In a food processor, grind your cookies.
4. Place the crumbs of cookies in the pan evenly.
5. In a medium bowl, mix the remaining ingredients together. Pour them in the crust and bake for about 45 minutes. To check if they're baked properly, see if a knife inserted in the middle comes out clean.
6. Allow it to cool and store in a refrigerator. Slice it into 8 wedges before serving.
Enjoy!

Strawberry Cheesecake

Ingredients
- 1 cup of sour cream
- 1/3 cup of sugar
- 8 ounces of softened cream cheese
- 8 ounces of whipped topping, prepared and thawed
- 2 teaspoons of pure vanilla extract
- One graham cracker crust of 6 ounces
- 1 pound of fresh strawberries, halved lengthwise and hulled

Instructions

1. Beat the cream cheese with an electric mixer until it's smooth. Slowly beat in the sugar followed by sour cream and vanilla and mix thoroughly. Fold in the topping and scrape the mixture into the crust. Chill the pie in a refrigerator for about 4 hours.

If there's extra filling, you can reserve it for decorating the top of the pie.

2. Arrange the strawberries in a circular pattern on top of the pie, starting with the middle.

Enjoy!

Side dishes

Asparagus & Horseradish

Nutrition per 2 asparagus spears with 1 Tbsp horseradish dip: Calories 63 – Fat 5 gr. – Sodium 146 mgr. – Carbs 3 gr. – Fiber – 0 gr. – Sugar 1 gr. – Protein 1 gr.

Ingredients
- 1 cup of mayonnaise, reduced-fat
- ¼ cup of Parmesan cheese, grated
- 1 Tbsp of prepared horseradish
- ½ tsp of Worcestershire sauce
- 32 (2 lbs.) asparagus spears, fresh and trimmed

Instructions
1. Take a steamer basket and put the asparagus in it. Then place it over one inch of water in a large saucepan. Steam the asparagus for about 2-4 minutes until it's crisp and tender.
2. Mix the rest of the ingredients in a small bowl and serve them with the asparagus.

Enjoy!

Baked Zucchini with Cheese

Serves: two
Nutrition per serving: Calories 64 – Fat 4 gr. – Sodium 85 mgr. – Carbs 4 gr. – Fiber 1 gr. – Sugar 2.5 gr. – Protein 3 gr.

Ingredients
- 1/8 tsp of garlic powder
- 1 tsp of olive oil
- 1/8 tsp of onion powder
- 2 Tbsp of Parmesan cheese, grated
- 1 zucchini (about 6" long)

Instructions
1. Heat the oven to 375 F.
2. Slice most of the zucchini after every half inch, but don't cut it all the way down. The slices must be held together. Trim it on its ends.
3. Pat it with a paper towel and place it on a foil. Drizzle some olive oil on top and sprinkle garlic powder and onion powder. Completely wrap the zucchini in the foil and place it on a baking sheet.
4. Place it in the oven and bake for about 30-35 minutes or until the zucchini is tender.
5. Sprinkle some cheese on top and leave the foil open. Now put it in the oven once again and bake for another 1-2 minutes to melt the cheese. Serve it warm. Enjoy!

Broccoli with Lemon

Serves: two

Nutrition per serving: Calories 45 – Fat 1 gr. – Sodium 153 mgr. – Carbs 7 gr. – Fiber 3 gr. – Sugar 2 gr. – Protein 3 gr.

Ingredients

- ¼ tsp of ground black pepper
- ¼ tsp of kosher salt
- 1 tsp of lemon zest
- 1 tsp of olive oil
- 1 Tbsp of minced garlic
- 4 cups of broccoli florets

Instructions

1. Boil a cup of water in a small saucepan. While the water is boiling, pour the broccoli in it and cook for about 2-3 minutes or until it's tender. Drain it.
2. Heat the heat over medium-high in a small sauté pan. Add garlic to it and sauté for about 30 seconds. Now add the remaining ingredients, mix them well and serve.

Enjoy!

Butternut Squash Fries

Serves: six

Nutrition per serving: Calories 62 – Fat 2 gr. – Sodium 168 mgr. – Carbs 11 gr. – Fiber 3 gr. – Sugar 2 gr. – Protein 1 gr.

Ingredients

- 1 Tbsp of fresh rosemary, chopped
- 1 Tbsp of fresh thyme, chopped
- 1 Tbsp of olive oil
- ½ tsp of salt
- 1 medium butternut squash

Instructions

1. Heat the oven to 425 F. Spray a baking sheet with some nonstick cooking spray.
2. Peel the butternut squash and cut it into pieces that are about 1/2" wide and 3" long.
3. In a medium bowl, mix the squash with oil, rosemary, thyme and salt until the squash is evenly coated.
4. Place it on the baking sheet and roast for about 10 minutes. Remove it from the oven and slightly shake the sheet to loosen the squash. Roast for another 5-10 minutes or until the squash turns golden-brown.

Enjoy!

Edamame Salad

Nutrition per serving: Calories 317 – Fat 17 gr. – Sodium 32 mgr. – Carbs 32 gr. – Fiber 8 gr. – Sugar 14 gr. – Protein 13 gr.

Ingredients

- 1 can of garbanzo beans (of 15 oz.) or chickpeas, drained and rinsed
- 6 cups of baby kale salad blend (5 oz.)
- 1 cup of bean sprouts, fresh
- ½ cup of salted peanuts
- ½ cup of sesame ginger salad dressing
- 2 cups of shelled edamame (about 10 oz.), frozen, thawed
- 3 clementines, peeled and segmented
- 2 green onions, sliced diagonally

Instructions

1. Place the salad blend evenly in 6 bowls.
2. Top the bowls with the remaining ingredients besides the salad dressing.
3. Serve it with the dressing.

Enjoy!

Tips:

- Edamame is Japanese for boiled or steamed green soybeans.
- Cutting the green onions slightly diagonally gives them an elegant look.

- *If clementines aren't available, use a navel orange.*
- *Clementines are rich in Vitamin C and can help your body absorb iron from plant sources.*

Cauliflower Mashed Potatoes

Serves: four

Nutrition per serving: Calories 67 – Fat 3 gr. – Sodium 60 mgr. – Carbs 9 gr. – Fiber 2.5 gr. – Sugar 3 gr. – Protein 2 gr.

Ingredients

- Head of a cauliflower
- 1 clove of garlic
- 1 white leek, split in four pieces
- 1 Tbsp of margarine (soft-tub), nonhydrogenated
- Pepper (to taste)

Instructions

1. Cut down the cauliflower into small pieces.
2. Steam the cauliflower along with garlic and leeks in water in a large saucepan for about 20-30 minutes.
3. Puree the vegetables in a food processor until they look like mashed potatoes. *You'll want to do this with a small portion at a time.*

You can also use a blender if you prefer a smoother texture. If you're using a blender, hold tightly onto the lid with a towel and add some water if the vegetables are dry.

4. Mix it with margarine and pepper.

Enjoy!

Lemon Rice with Raisins & Almonds

Serves: four

Nutrition per serving: Calories 200 – Fat 5 gr. – Sodium 66 mgr. – Carbs 34 gr. – Fiber 3 gr. – Sugar 4 gr. – Protein 4 gr.

Ingredients

- 1 cup of brown rice, uncooked
- 1 ¾ cups of chicken broth, unsalted
- 1 cup of frozen peas
- ½ cup of golden raisins
- ¼ cup of onions, chopped
- ½ cup of slivered almonds, chopped coarsely
- 1/3 cups of water
- 2 Tbsp of honey
- 3 Tbsp of lemon juice
- 1 Tbsp of trans-fat margarine
- ½ tsp of ground cinnamon
- ¼ tsp of ground nutmeg
- 2 tsp of lemon zest

Instructions

1. Preheat the oven to 325 F. Lightly spray a baking sheet with nonstick cooking spray.
2. Place the almonds on the sheet and bake for about 10 minutes, stirring occasionally, until they're golden. Allow them to cool in a plate.
3. Add the lemon juice, lemon zest, broth, cinnamon, rice, onions, nutmeg and margarine in the top section of a double boiler. In the bottom of the

boiler, add water. Heat the boiler and stir occasionally. Cover it and let it simmer for about 30 minutes.

4.   Add water and raisins to a small saucepan, and simmer and cook for about 5 minutes. Now add in the peas and simmer for one more minute. Add this mixture to the rice mix in the double boiler and simmer for about 15-20 minutes or more, so that the liquid gets absorbed.

5.   Mix the rice mixture and place it on a serving dish. Sprinkle the toasted almonds and drizzle some honey on top.

Enjoy!

Minted Carrots

Serves: six

Nutrition per serving: Calories 44 – Fat trace – Sodium 51 mgr. – Carbs 10 gr. – Fiber 2.5 gr. – Sugar 5 gr. – Protein 1 gr.

Ingredients

- 1 lb. of rinsed baby carrots
- 1 cup of apple juice
- 6 cups of water
- 1 Tbsp of cornstarch
- ½ Tbsp of mint leaves, fresh and chopped
- 1/8 tsp of ground cinnamon

Instructions

1. Add water and carrots in a large sized pan and boil for about 10 minutes. Drain the carrots and place them in a bowl to serve.
2. Mix the apple juice and cornstarch over medium heat in a small saucepan. Stir the mixture for about 5 minutes, until it thickens. Now add and stir the cinnamon and mint.
3. Add the mixture onto the carrots.

Enjoy!

Quinoa Peppers

Nutrition per 1 cup: Calories 261 – Fat 9 gr. – Sodium 760 mgr. – Carbs 28 gr. – Fiber 4 gr. – Sugar 3 gr. – Protein 17 gr.

Ingredients

- 1 ½ cups of vegetable stock
- ¾ cups of rinsed quinoa
- ¾ cups of sweet onion, chopped
- 1 lb. of Italian turkey sausage links (remove their casings)
- 1 medium chopped green pepper
- 1 medium chopped sweet red pepper
- 1 minced garlic clove
- ¼ tsp of garam masala
- ¼ tsp of pepper
- 1/8 tsp of salt

Instructions

1. Boil the vegetable stock in a small saucepan. Add to it the quinoa and decrease the heat. Cover it and simmer for about 12-15 minutes, until the liquid gets absorbed. Set it aside.
2. Crumble and cook the sausage with onions and peppers (about 8-10 minutes) in large skillet over medium-high heat. Mix garlic and seasonings and cook for about 1 more minute while stirring. Stir the quinoa with the mixture.

To Freeze: put them in freezer containers and refrigerate overnight. Microwave them on high setting.

Enjoy!

Tip: *You could also use chicken or beef stock in place of vegetable stock.*

Green Beans, Roasted

Serves: four

Nutrition per serving: Calories 59 – Fat 3 gr. – Sodium 132 mgr. – Carbs 9 gr. – Fiber 3 gr. – Sugar 4 gr. – Protein 2 gr.

Ingredients

- 1 cup of cherry tomatoes
- 2 cups of cleaned and trimmed green beans
- 1 Tbsp of minced garlic
- 1 tsp of dried basil
- 1 tsp of dried oregano
- 2 tsp of olive oil
- 1 tsp of onion powder
- ½ tsp of pepper
- ½ tsp of salt

Instructions

1. Heat the oven to 400 F.
2. In a medium bowl, mix the basil, green beans, tomatoes, oil, garlic, oregano, onion powder, salt and pepper, until the beans are well mixed with olive oil and seasoning.
3. Lightly grease a baking sheet and spread the beans evenly onto it. Roast in the oven for about 10-15 minutes and stir them after 10 minutes.

Enjoy!

Sautéed Corn

Serves: six

Nutrition per serving: Calories 78 – Fat 2 gr. – Sodium 216 mgr. – Carbs 11 gr. – Fiber 1 gr. – Sugar 4 gr. – Protein 4 gr.

Ingredients

- 2 cups of corn kernels, fresh (obtained from about four medium ears of corn) or frozen corn
- 1 seeded, cored and diced green bell pepper
- 1 tsp of olive oil
- 1 tsp of minced garlic
- 2 oz. of prosciutto (thin strips of it)

Instructions

- Heat the olive oil over medium heat in a large sized skillet. Pour in the prosciutto and sauté for about 5 minutes, until it's crisp. Mix and stir the bell pepper, corn and garlic and sauté for about 5-7 minutes while stirring occasionally.

Enjoy!

Fried Endive

Serves: four

Nutrition per serving: Calories 24 – Fat: trace – Sodium 150 mgr. – Carbs 5 gr. – Fiber 3 gr. – Sugar (added) 0 gr. – Protein 1 gr.

Ingredients

- 8 washed and halved heads of Belgian endive
- Juice of one lemon
- 1 Tbsp of water
- 2 Tbsp of fresh parsley, chopped
- ½ tsp of salt
- Ground black pepper (optional for taste)

Instructions

1. Heat the water over medium heat in a large skillet and mix the endives in it (with its cut sides facing down). Cook it while keeping it covered until its outer leaves are translucent.
2. Set it aside and pour the lemon juice, salt and pepper to taste.
3. Place it on a serving dish and use parsley as garnishing. Serve it.

Enjoy!

Sweet Potatoes & Bananas

Serves: six

Nutrition per serving: Calories 156 – Fat: trace – Sodium 64 mgr. – Carbs 37 gr. – Fiber 5 gr. – Sugar (added) 4 gr. – Protein 2 gr.

Ingredients

- 2 peeled and halved medium bananas
- 1 ½ lbs. of washed sweet potatoes
- 2 Tbsp of orange juice
- ¼ tsp of ground cardamom
- ½ tsp of ground cinnamon
- ¼ tsp of ground nutmeg
- 3 Tbsp of brown sugar
- Red pepper flakes (to taste)
- Parsley, chopped (for garnish)

Instructions

1. Heat the oven to 375 F. Spray some nonstick cooking spray on a baking dish.
2. Make holes with a fork in the sweet potatoes and place them in the oven. Bake for about 1 hour until they're soft. Set them aside and peel them once they're cool.
3. Add the banana halves to the baking dish and bake for about 15 minutes until the bananas are juicy and soft. Remove them from the oven and mix them with orange juice. Stir and mash the bananas.

4. Add the bananas, brown sugar, spices and sweet potatoes in a large mixing bowl and blend them with an electric mixer until they give a smooth consistency.
5. Bake them in the oven until they're warm in an ovenproof bowl.
6. Use the parsley as garnish and serve.
Enjoy!

Warm Coleslaw

Serves: six

Nutrition per serving: Calories 74 – Fat 5 gr. – Sodium 117 mgr. – Carbs 8 gr. – Fiber 2 gr. – Sugar (added) 3 gr. – Protein 1 gr.

Ingredients

- 1 finely chopped, medium yellow onion (~ ½ cup)
- 1 peel and julienned large carrot (~ 1 cup)
- ½ cored and thinly sliced head of Napa cabbage (~ 5 cups)
- 1 tsp of dry mustard
- 6 tsp of olive oil
- 1 Tbsp of Italian parsley, fresh and chopped
- 3 Tbsp of cider vinegar
- 1 Tbsp of dark honey
- ¼ tsp of black pepper, freshly ground
- ½ tsp of caraway seed
- ¼ tsp of salt

Instructions

1. Heat the olive oil over medium-high flame in a large sized nonstick sauté pan. Mix the onion and mustard in it and sauté for about 6 minutes until the onion turns tender and light golden in color. Place the mixture in a large bowl.

2. Add two more tsp of olive oil to the pan and put it over medium heat. Add the carrot, tossing and stirring it for about 3 minutes, until it's tender and crisp. Mix it with the onion mixture.

3.   Add the remaining oil to the pan and put it over medium heat. Add the cabbage, tossing and stirring it for about 3 minutes. Then transfer the cabbage to bowl of carrots and onion mixture.

4.   Without wasting any time, add the honey and vinegar to the pan over medium heat and stir until they're thoroughly mixed and bubbly and the honey is dissolved. Pour the coleslaw on top and mix it with salt and pepper, tossing them well so they're thoroughly combined.

5.   Use caraway seed and parsley as garnish and serve warm.

Enjoy!

Extras: chips, dips and more

Dash Artichoke Dip

Serves: eight

Nutrition per serving: Calories 78 – Fat 2 gr. – Sodium 130 mgr. – Carbs 10 gr. – Fiber 6 gr. – Sugar 1.5 gr. – Protein 5 gr.

Ingredients

- 2 cloves of minced garlic
- 1 (15.5 oz.) can of artichoke hearts in water, drained
- ½ cup of low-fat sour cream
- 4 cups of raw spinach, chopped
- 1 cup of white beans, prepared and unsalted
- 1 tsp of ground black pepper
- 1 tsp of minced fresh thyme (or 1/3 tsp of dried fresh thyme)
- 1 Tbsp of fresh minced parsley (or 1 tsp of dried parsley)
- 2 Tbsp of grated Parmesan cheese

Instructions

- Mix all ingredients in a mixing bowl and place in a ceramic dish. Bake at 350 F for about 30 minutes. Enjoy!

Bean Hummus

Ingredients

- 1 clove of garlic or 1/8 tsp of garlic powder
- 1 cup of garbanzo beans, cooked and drained
- 2 Tbsp of lemon juice
- ¼ tsp of black pepper
- ½ tsp of ground cumin
- 2 tsp of vegetable oil or olive oil
- ½ cup of nonfat plain yogurt

Instructions

Method 1:
1. Blend all ingredients in a blender for your desired consistency (smooth or chunky).
2. Add 2 teaspoons of water if the hummus is too thick for your taste and refrigerate the leftovers within 2 hours.

Method 2:
- Place the beans on a large plate and mash them with a fork until they're smooth.
- In a small bowl, mix the beans with the rest of the ingredients.
- Add 2 teaspoons of water if the hummus is too thick for your taste and refrigerate the leftovers within 2 hours.

Enjoy!

Cornmeal Muffins

Servings: twelve muffins

Nutrition per serving: Calories 120 – Fat < 1 gr. – Sodium 128 mgr. – Carbs 26 gr. – Fiber 1 gr. – Sugar 7 gr. – Protein 4 gr.

Ingredients

- 1 cored, peeled and coarsely chopped apple
- 2 egg whites
- 2 cups of all-purpose flour
- ¼ cup of brown sugar, packed
- ¾ cups of milk (fat-free)
- ½ cup of fresh or frozen corn kernels
- ½ cup of yellow cornmeal
- 1 Tbsp of baking powder
- ¼ tsp of salt

Instructions

1. Heat the oven to 425 F.
2. Line a muffin pan (12 cup) with foil. You can also use paper liners.
3. Stir and blend evenly the baking powder, brown sugar, cornmeal, flour and salt in a large sized bowl.
4. Mix the egg whites with milk in a small bowl and add the apple and corn kernels. Whisk it and pour it over the flour mixture. Now stir gently (the dry ingredients should be lightly moist) and the batter should have a lumpy consistency.
5. Fill two thirds of the cups with the mixture and bake for about 30 minutes.

Enjoy!

Potato Skins

Serves: two

Nutrition per serving: Calories 114 – Fat 0 gr. – Sodium 18 mgr. – Carbs 27 gr. – Fiber 5 gr. – Sugar (added) 0 gr. – Protein 2 gr.

Ingredients

- Cooking spray (butter flavored)
- Two medium russet potatoes
- 1/8 tsp of freshly ground black pepper
- 1 Tbsp of minced fresh rosemary

Instructions

1. Preheat the oven to 375 F.
2. Wash the potatoes and cut them with a fork. Put them in the oven and bake for about an hour, until they're crisp.
3. Cut the potatoes in half (very carefully as they'll be hot) and scoop out their pulp, and make sure 1/8" of the flesh is still attached to the skin. You'll use the pulp for a later time.
4. Spray the cooking spray inside of each potato skin and tuck in the rosemary and pepper.
5. Place the skins in the oven and bake for about 5-10 minutes.

Enjoy!

Guacamole & Beans

Serves: eight

Nutrition per serving: Calories 59 – Fat 3 gr. – Sodium 25 mgr. – Carbs 6 gr. – Fiber 3 gr. – Sugar 0.5 gr. – Protein 2 gr.

Ingredients

- ½ cup of canned black or pinto beans (no salt added), drained and rinsed
- 1 diced avocado (~ ½ cup)
- 1 large diced ripe tomato (~ 1 cup)
- Juice of one lime (~ 2 Tbsp)
- Optional: ¼ tsp of cayenne, chipotle or ancho chili powder
- 2 tsp of ground cumin
- ¼ cup of shallot, chopped

Instructions

- Combine the avocado, beans, cayenne pepper, cumin and lime juice in a medium bowl. Blend them with the shallot and tomato.

Enjoy!

Brown Bread (Irish)

Serves: twenty-four
Nutrition per serving: Calories 85 – Fat 1 gr. – Sodium 170 mgr. – Carbs 15 gr. – Fiber 1.5 gr. – Sugar 1 gr. – Protein 4 gr.

Ingredients

- 1 ½ cups of all-purpose flour
- 2 cups of buttermilk, low-fat
- ½ cup of wheat germ
- 2 cups of flour (whole-wheat)
- 2 tsp of baking soda
- ¼ tsp of salt
- 1 lightly beaten egg

Instructions

1. Heat the oven to 400 F and prepare a nonstick baking sheet.
2. Mix and whisk to blend the flours in a bowl along with baking soda, salt and wheat germ. Mix the egg and buttermilk in it and stir — the dough will have a sticky consistency.
3. Put some flour on a clean surface for kneading the dough and apply the flour on your hands. Now gently knead the dough for about 8-10 minutes. It should form a ball shape.
4. Place the dough on the baking sheet and mold it into a 7" round shape. Apply a small amount of flour on the top to dust it. Now cut an approximately 4" X on the top of the dough (about 1/2" deep).

5. Bake for about 25-30 minutes until the bread opens at the X. Before you slice it, allow it to cool on a wire rack for about 2 hours.
Enjoy!

Kale Chips

Ingredients
- 2 tsp of olive oil
- 1 bunch of kale

Instructions
1. Preheat the oven to 200 F. Spray vegetable oil cooking spray on 2 large baking sheets.
2. Wash and fully dry the kale.
3. Remove the leaves from stems and the rib in the middle of the leaves. Then cut it into large sections.
4. In a large bowl, pour 1 tsp of olive oil and mix it thoroughly with the kale.
5. Place it evenly in a single layer on each baking sheet.
6. Bake for about 20 minutes and turn the chips over.
7. Bake for about 10 more minutes, or until they're crisp.
8. Allow the chips to cool on a cooling rack. Place them in a bowl and sprinkle with grated Parmesan cheese or salt, if you so desire.
Enjoy!

Sweet Potato Chips

Ingredients
- A dash of olive oil
- A pinch of sea salt
- Two sweet potatoes

Instructions

1. Slice the potatoes thin. Drizzle with olive oil and sprinkle some sea salt on top.
2. Bake in a microwave on high setting for about 2-3 minutes until they turn brown.
3. Flip them over and microwave again.

Enjoy!

Spicy Tortilla Chips

Ingredients

- Nonstick spray oil
- Corn tortillas, soft
- Spices of your choosing

Instructions

1. Cut the tortillas in quarters. You can use flour tortillas too, but keep in mind that the fat and sodium levels will increase quite a lot.

2. Place them on a baking sheet and spray them with the nonstick spray oil. Sprinkle the seasoning of your choice.

3. Bake at 400 F for about 6-10 minutes or until they're crispy.

Enjoy!

Dash Vegetable Salsa

Serves: sixteen

Nutrition per serving: Calories 24 – Fat 0 gr. – Sodium 79 mgr. – Carbs 5 gr. – Fiber 1 gr. – Sugar 2 gr. – Protein 1 gr.

Ingredients

- ½ cup of fresh cilantro, chopped
- ¼ cup of lime juice
- 1 cup of red onion, chopped
- 1 cup of zucchini, diced
- 2 seeded and diced green bell peppers (~ 2 cups)
- 2 seeded and diced red bell peppers (~ 2 cups)
- 4 diced tomatoes (~ 2 cups)
- 2 cloves of minced garlic
- 1 tsp of ground black pepper
- ½ tsp of salt
- 2 tsp of sugar

Instructions

1. Wash and prepare the vegetables.
2. Pour and toss all ingredients in a large bowl, so that they're mixed thoroughly.
3. Refrigerate the mixture covered for about 30 minutes for the flavors to blend.

Enjoy!

Bean Dip

Serves: eight

Nutrition per serving: Calories 84 – Fat 4 gr. – Sodium 123 mgr. – Carbs 9 gr. – Fiber 3 gr. – Sugar (added) 0 gr. – Protein 3 gr.

Ingredients

- 8 roasted cloves of garlic
- 1 (15 oz.) can of white cannellini beans, rinsed and drained
- 2 Tbsp of lemon juice
- 2 Tbsp of olive oil

Instructions

1. Blend the beans, roasted garlic, lemon juice and olive oil in a blender or food processor. The mixture should be smooth.
2. Layer the mixture on top of thin slices of toasted French bread (you can also use pita triangles).
3. This is optional, but it also goes splendidly well when placed on top of sweet red bell peppers (cut in squares).

Enjoy!

Dash Whole Wheat Pretzels

Serves: fourteen

Nutrition per serving: Calories 148 – Fat 2 gr. – Sodium 76 mgr. – Carbs 27 gr. – Fiber 3 gr. – Sugar 1 gr. – Protein 8 gr.

Ingredients

- ¼ cup of baking soda
- 1 cup of bread flour
- 1 ½ cups of warm water
- ½ cup of wheat gluten
- 3 cups of whole wheat flour
- 1 pack of dry active yeast
- 2 tsp of brown sugar
- ½ tsp of kosher salt
- 1 Tbsp of olive oil
- 1 Tbsp of sesame, sunflower or poppy seeds
- Cooking spray
- 1 egg white (or ¼ cup of egg substitute)

Instructions

1. Mix salt, sugar, yeast in warm water in a food processor bowl, and let it sit for about 5 minutes. Now add in the flours, gluten and olive oil and mix for about 5-10 minutes (you can mix by hand or in the food processor with a dough hook). A smooth dough should form.

2. Spray nonstick cooking spray in the bowl so that the dough doesn't stick. Wrap a plastic cover on top

and set it aside for about 1 hour or until it doubles in size.

3. Make 14 pieces of the dough by punching it down and roll these to form long ropes. Make each rope into a U-shape. Now pinch at the bottom of the U-shape and cross its ends over to make a pretzel shape.

4. Boil 8-10 cups of water with ¼ cup of baking soda and cook the pretzels for about 30 minutes.

5. Line a baking pan with parchment paper and place the pretzels on it. Gently brush them with the egg white and add your choice of seasoning on top.

6. Bake in an oven at 450 F for about 10-15 minutes.

Enjoy!

Dash Zucchini Bread

Serves: eighteen

Nutrition per serving: Calories 141 – Fat 5 gr. – Sodium 103 mgr. – Carbs 22 gr. – Fiber 2 gr. – Sugar (added) 5 gr. – Protein 4 gr.

Ingredients

- 1 ¼ cups of all-purpose flour (plain)
- ½ cup of applesauce, unsweetened
- ¼ cup of canola oil
- 1 ½ cups of pineapple, crushed and unsweetened
- ½ cup of sugar
- ½ cup of walnuts, chopped
- 1 ¼ cups of whole-wheat flour
- 2 cups of zucchini, shredded
- 6 egg whites
- 1 tsp of baking powder
- 1 tsp of baking soda
- 3 tsp of ground cinnamon
- 2 tsp of vanilla extract

Instructions

1. Heat the oven to 350 F.
2. Spray two 9x5" loaf pans cooking spray.
3. Beat the applesauce, canola oil, egg whites, sugar and vanilla in a large bowl using an electric mixer on low speed until the mixture is thick.
4. Stir the flours together in a small bowl and set ½ cup aside. To the flour bowl, add the baking powder, baking soda and cinnamon.

5.   Pour this mixture in the egg mixture and beat with an electric mixer on medium speed. Mix and stir in the pineapple, walnuts and zucchini. Make the resulting batter thick in consistency by adding the ½ cup of flour, one tablespoon at a time.
6.   Pour half of the batter into each loaf pan and bake for about 50 minutes. Allow the bread to cool on a wire rack for about 10 minutes. Take the loaves out of the pans and allow them to cool fully.
7.   Cut each loaf into nine 1" slices.
Enjoy!

Zucchini Parmesan Chips

Ingredients

- 3 washed, medium zucchini squash with their ends trimmed
- 1 egg white (large)
- ¼ cup of grated parmesan cheese
- 2 tablespoons of parsley flakes, dried
- 1 ½ teaspoon of Dill weed seasoning
- 1 teaspoon of garlic powder
- 1 teaspoon of onion powder
- ¼ teaspoon of pepper (or to taste)
- ¼ teaspoon of salt (or to taste)

Instructions

1. Preheat the oven to 425 F.
2. Line a baking sheet with foil and spray it with cooking spray.
3. Cut the zucchini into 1/8" disks having approximately the same thickness so that they'll cook evenly.
4. Whisk the egg white in a medium sized bowl and add and toss the zucchini in it so that they're coated evenly.
5. In a large sized Ziplock bag, add the parmesan cheese and seasoning mixture and shake them well to combine. Add the zucchini to the bag and shake it well to coat the zucchini with the seasoning.
6. Lay the zucchini chips onto the baking pan and bake for about 25-30 minutes. Also, broil on high heat

for about 1-2 minutes (or until the coating is crisp and light brown in color).
7. Take it off from the oven and serve it warm with your choice of dip.
Enjoy!

Part 2

Introduction

Welcome to the DASH Diet! You are starting a journey, which will change your relationship with food forever. In doing so, you are choosing a lifestyle where you are fully nourishing your body and optimizing your health, without completely giving up the foods you love.

Going on the DASH Diet is one of the healthiest lifestyle choices you can make. And with a little guidance and preparation, you can easily transform your eating habits to lower your blood pressure, lose weight, and guard against health risks and disease. The DASH Diet is your path to feeling good, everyday.

With a little preparation, the DASH Diet is easy to follow and maintain. This book simplifies the DASH Diet so you can easily understand the benefits, see how it works, and gain insight into preparing meals, snacks, and exercise routines.

Beyond the methodology of the DASH Diet, this book offers meal plans and delicious recipes to make everything simple! As you will see, some of the recipes are meals and snacks you can throw together quick for those days when you just don't have time, and some are wholesome meals when you have time for something extraordinary.

Additionally, this book offers easy-to-follow tips to make everything as simple as possible. These tips will get you started the right way and help keep you on track until the DASH Diet is second-nature to you.

Lastly, you will find 20 recipes to get you through the first two weeks of the DASH Diet. As we'll discuss, the first two weeks of the DASH Diet are different than the regular program, but you'll find these recipes are easy to adapt and give you a wide variety of foods. Also, the recipes include breakfast, lunch, dinner, and dessert.

Keep in mind, if you want to lose weight and keep it off, it takes some work. But the DASH Diet offers a plan that will put you on track for a healthy lifestyle, that's easy to maintain, and will change the way you think about food.

Following this plan is a ticket to healthy lifestyle. So let's get to it!

Chapter 1: the dash diet basics: lowering blood pressure and losing weight

"DASH" stands for Dietary Approaches to Stop Hypertension. It is a food and nutrition plan that was first developed to treat patients with hypertension (more commonly known as high blood pressure). It is designed to lower blood pressure by reducing sodium intake.

After research showed that high blood pressure was much less prevalent in people who ate vegetarian and vegan diets, researchers sought to develop a diet that reduced sodium and provided generous amounts of nutrients that protect people against high blood pressure.

The result was a diet that prioritizes fruits and vegetables, and includes generous amounts of low-fat and nonfat dairy, whole grains, and lean proteins like poultry, fish, and beans. It is well-rounded with a full variety of foods, and while it is low in red meat, salt, sugar, and saturated fat, it does not eliminate any food groups.

Additionally, the diet recommends nutrient-rich food sources to achieve daily-recommended amounts of vitamins and minerals; especially those that help reduce blood pressure. These vitamins include magnesium, calcium, and potassium.

Although the purpose of the DASH Diet was to reduce blood pressure, researchers found that people who followed the diet were also losing weight as a side effect. With a few minor adjustments, people who follow the DASH Diet can easily and efficiently lose weight and keep it off. This has made the DASH Diet one of the most popular and top-rated diets today.

Furthermore, the DASH Diet is highly supported by doctors and other health professionals, and the National Heart, Lung & Blood Institute and The American Heart Association endorse it. The US Departments of Agriculture and Health and Human Services Dietary Guidelines for Americans states that the DASH Diet is in line with their guidelines.

By following the DASH Diet, you will lower your blood pressure and lose weight, but you will also achieve additional health benefits including the following:

- Protection against heart disease and stroke: Following the DASH diet lowers homocysteine levels and LDL cholesterols, which are thought to contribute to plaque build-up on artery walls and increase the risk of heart disease and stroke.
- Improved insulin resistance: The DASH diet includes high amounts of calcium, magnesium, and fiber, and low amounts of saturated fat, which have been found to improve insulin resistance for individuals with type 2 diabetes.
- Cholesterol problems: The DASH Diet helps to reduce bad cholesterol and increase good cholesterol, which is necessary for the body.

- All day energy: The DASH Diet helps regulate blood sugar and provide the daily-recommended amounts of nutrients, helping avoid peaks and crashes, and keeping your body more energized during the course of a day.

Overall, the DASH Diet is considered to be one of the healthiest diets you could choose. DASH isn't just for people with high blood pressure; it's a healthy, wholesome, high-fiber eating plan than can also help improve cholesterol levels and promote weight loss. Furthermore, it is designed as a method of eating that you can maintain for a lifetime.

High blood pressure and the DASH Diet solution

The DASH Diet was originally developed to treat or prevent hypertension, so it's important to understand what hypertension is, and why it matters.

Hypertension, more commonly called high blood pressure, is when the force of blood against the artery walls is consistently higher than normal. The elevated force is the result of build-up along artery walls, which narrows the space that blood flows through. The narrower the space, the harder your heart has to work to move blood around your body, hence the increase in pressure.

High blood pressure can lead to a host of medical problems and risks including: heart attack or failure, stroke, aneurysms, metabolic syndrome, chronic kidney disease, coronary artery disease, vision loss, memory problems, and damage to blood vessels and to various organs.

The United States has seen a significant increase in high blood pressure, in the last 50 years. According to the Centers for Disease Control and Prevention, about 75 million American adults, meaning 1 out of 3, have high blood pressure. (https://www.cdc.gov/bloodpressure/facts.htm)

Certain factors increase the risk for high blood pressure including: age (over 45 for men, over 65 for women), family history, being overweight or obese, not being physically active, stress, smoking or chewing tobacco, certain medical conditions, and having a high salt, low potassium, or low vitamin D diet.

High blood pressure generally develops over a long period of time. You could have high blood pressure for years, causing damage to blood vessels, and your heart could continue without any symptoms. Even though most people do not present with symptoms from high blood pressure, it is easy to detect. You will likely have your blood pressure taken as part of a routine doctors appointment. If you don't see a doctor regularly, you can ask for a test at a local clinic.

A blood pressure reading has two numbers. For example, a normal blood pressure reading is below 120/80 mm Hg (read 120 over 80). The top number measures the blood pressure when your heart beats. This is called systolic pressure. The bottom number measures the blood pressure between heartbeats. This is called diastolic pressure.

Blood pressure is categorized as either normal, prehypertension, stage 1 hypertension, or stage 2 hypertension.

The readings for each category is as follows:

Normal blood pressure is below 120/80 mm Hg.

Prehypertension means systolic pressure ranges from 120 to 139 mm Hg or a diastolic pressure ranges from 80 to 89 mm Hg.

Stage 1 hypertension means systolic pressure ranges from 140 to 159 mm Hg or a diastolic pressure ranges from 90 to 99 mm Hg.

Stage 2 hypertension means there is a systolic pressure of 160 mm Hg or higher or a diastolic pressure of 100 mm Hg or higher.

Diet plays a major role in the development of high blood pressure. Dietary changes made by following the DASH Diet can help lower blood pressure and protect against the health risks caused by high blood pressure. Additionally, the DASH Diet is an effective way to lose weight and keep it off.

The DASH Diet and weight loss

The DASH Diet was not designed as a weight-loss program. However, since it is a well-rounded, healthy diet, research has shown that people who followed the diet typically lost weight.

When following the DASH Diet, you consume about 2,000 calories a day. If you are trying to lose weight on the diet, you can simply lower your calorie intake, increase your physical activity, or reset your metabolism with a low-carb, low sugar phase.

Marla Heller, the dietitian responsible for bringing the DASH Diet to the general public through several books, recommends a two-phase plan to getting the body on track for weight loss using the DASH Diet.

By adding a two-week, low-carb and low sugar phase to reset metabolism, and by making some minor adjustments in one's regular routine, the DASH Diet easily becomes a healthy and effective weight-loss program. It is also a long-term strategy for maintaining a healthy weight.

Chapter 2: the dash diet: how it works

Like most diets, the DASH Diet requires some planning and preparation. To be successful, you have to plan-out weekly meals, create grocery lists, and make time to prepare or cook meals each day. At the beginning, you will also want to check nutrition labels for calories, fat content, vitamins, minerals, and protein. In later chapters, you will find a meal plan and recipes to help guide you, but you will want to make adjustments to meet your personal needs.

Despite the need to prepare, the DASH Diet is easy to follow because it allows a wide variety of food choices and the program is easy to understand. Also, the DASH Diet does not eliminate any food groups, so you can avoid cravings and never feel like you have to miss out on the foods you love.

Types of DASH Diets

There are three versions of the DASH Diet: the original DASH Diet for lowering blood pressure, the weight loss plan, and the vegetarian plan.

In this book, we focus on the weight loss plan and by doing so, we will cover all three DASH Diets. The weight loss plan consists of two phases. The first phase is a two-week, low-carb, low sugar regiment to reset your metabolism and train your body to feel full from eating proper amounts of protein, nutrients, and healthy fats. Phase two of the weight loss plan is to follow the original DASH Diet. And you can do that for the rest of your life! Easy, right?

Finally, to understand the vegetarian DASH Diet plan, we will simply review the vegetable substitutes for meat and fish in the original plan. With that, you will be well-versed in all variations of the DASH Diet.

Two Phases of the DASH Diet

Phase one is a two-week, low-carb, low sugar diet that helps reset metabolism. During the first two weeks, you will increase lean proteins while eliminating fruits, starchy vegetables, and whole grains.

The components of phase one are: high protein, low-fat foods like fish, poultry, beans, soy, eggs, and low-fat dairy; moderate portions at meals; small snacks; and foods containing healthy and polyunsaturated fats such as avocado, nuts, vegetable oils, salmon, and mackerel.

Phase two will be the standard DASH Diet food and nutrition regiment, which you can follow indefinitely. You simply introduce the recommend amounts of fruits, starchy vegetables, and whole grains, while maintaining the recommended daily serving sizes.

The DASH Diet recommends focusing on eating specific types of food, such as vegetables (which are rich in nutrients), lean proteins, and healthy fats. With these foods, you will feel full and energized.

In addition to the low-carb, low-sugar phase, adding daily physical activity to your routine will help increase weight loss, as well as maintain it.

DASH Diet: Phase 1

Many people have trouble losing weight because spikes in blood sugar can lead to cravings and overeating. In Phase 1, the first two weeks of your DASH Diet, you will learn to focus on consuming foods that are high in fiber, protein, nutrients, and healthy fats that will make you feel full and energized.

Regulating blood sugar helps prevent cravings that often lead to overeating of carbs and sugar. By avoiding high carb, starchy, and sugary foods, you can help regulate your blood sugar. This means avoiding fruits and whole grains because they are high in sugar and carbs.

During Phase 1, you will focus heavily on dark, leafy greens like spinach and broccoli. You can have an unlimited amount of non-starchy vegetables; 2-4 servings of low-fat dairy per day; 2-4 servings of lean meats, fish, or poultry; 1-4 servings per day of healthy fats; and 1-2 servings of nuts, beans, and seeds. A serving size of cooked lean meat, poultry, or fish is 3 ounces. A good reference is 3 ounces of meat is about the same size as a deck of cards. Your dairy intake could be 1 cup of skim milk or low-fat yogurt per serving. As part of your plan, try to get your daily intake of healthy fats from foods like avocado, olive oil, and salmon.

DASH Diet: Phase 2

Phase 2 is essentially the original DASH Diet. It is a food and nutrition plan you can use to maintain a healthy lifestyle for the rest of your life. It focuses on appropriate daily servings of a variety of foods and low sodium intake to maintain a healthy blood pressure.

In Phase 2, you can eat the same foods as in Phase 1, but you will reintroduce fruits and whole grains, and you will adjust the serving sizes for the other food groups. Specifically, you will be eating 6 to 8 servings of whole grains and 4 to 5 servings of fruit each day. You will also eat 4-5 servings of vegetables; 2-3 servings of low-fat dairy; 6-11 servings of lean meats, poultry, or fish; and 2-3 servings of healthy fats every day. And each week you can have 4-5 servings of nuts, seeds, or beans and 5 or less servings of sugary sweets.

However, it's best to add fruits and whole grains gradually once you start. Start Phase 2 by adding 3 servings of whole grains and 2 servings of fruit. Then add a serving of each every few days until you reach your daily amounts.

In Phase 2, no food groups are off-limits. You can eat fruits, vegetables, low-fat dairy, lean meats, fish, poultry, legumes, nuts, seeds, and a little bit of fat and sweets.

Instead of cutting out certain food groups, it's important to regulate how much of each food group you eat, and always reach for foods that are low in salt and saturated fats first. In other words, you will want to continue to eat a variety of vegetables including plenty of dark, leafy greens, low-fat dairy, lean meats, fish, poultry, beans, and lentils.

Additionally, you will want to choose foods that are high in calcium, protein, and fiber. These foods help maintain a healthy blood pressure and keep you feeling satisfied.

During Phase 2, you can continue to lose weight gradually until you reach your goal. Then you can maintain your healthy weight and blood pressure by continuing to follow the DASH Diet lifestyle. Depending on your body, you may lose weight just by making the healthy change to the DASH Diet—you be eating better foods and getting more nutrients that make your body function more efficiently. For others, maybe cutting down the calories, adding a little more exercise, or a little of both will do the trick. Regardless, whatever your body needs, the DASH Diet will deliver.

A Few Tips Before We Begin

First step:

Figure out how many calories you need to consume each day and how many you burn during your exercise routines. Then determine how many servings you can eat from each food group based on those calories. In chapters below, you will find tools to help you determine these numbers.

Make a detailed meal plan and grocery list:

Once you know how many servings of each food group you can eat, you will be able to sit down and plan out your meals. The more prepared you are, the more likely you are to succeed. After a while, you'll get used to meal-types and portion sizes so it won't require much thought, but at the beginning, planning is essential.

Prepare your ingredients:

You should always prepare the required ingredients in advance to avoid last minute mistakes or missed meals.

Reward:

When you've reached your weekly goal, reward yourself. The best option is to choose a non-food reward. Do something you love as a way to celebrate your positive dietary changes.

Basic Mistakes to Avoid

Excessive Calorie Deficit:

We all do it. Any time we want to lose weight and get in shape, we want to see results as fast as possible. When trying to lose weight fast you can work out extra hard, eat way fewer calories, or both. The problem is, while you will lose weight quickly, it is likely you will gain it back.

Don't make this mistake; keep your long-term goal in mind. Any successful weight loss program relies on gradual weight loss, and on this point, the DASH Diet is no different. If you want to lose weight and keep it off, the best method is gradual weight loss with only a slight calorie deficit.

Avoiding Fats:

It is important to avoid saturated fats that raise bad cholesterol and increase risk of heart disease. However, fats help your body absorb essential vitamins and maintain proper body function. Therefore, it's important not to shy away from fats while following the DASH Diet; just opt for good fats – such as olive oil or avocado. The right amount of fats will depend on your daily calories (see below), but generally you should aim for about 2-3 servings of fat each day.

Lacking variety:

To achieve the best results, the DASH Diet recommends a wide variety of foods. This will not only ensure you are consuming all the necessary vitamins, but also that you aren't getting bored with the food you are eating. If you get sick of eating the same things, you're likely to crave unhealthy, carb-heavy or sweet foods. Get in the habit of seeking out and trying new, healthy recipes. Make eating healthy fun!

Chapter 3: know your calories

Unlike many diets, the DASH Diet does not focus on counting calories. However, before you start, you should have an idea of what your daily caloric intake should be. You can use this number to determine the amount of servings you should eat in each food group daily. Once you know how many servings of each food group you should eat and what the servicing size is, planning your meals will be much easier.

How many calories you need each day is largely based on weight, gender, age, and activity level. For now we are going to ignore activity level, but I'll explain why later.

First, figure out how many calories you should be taking in everyday. There are a few different ways to determine this amount. For example, you could just Google "how many calories should I eat" and you will find a bunch of calorie calculators. But you can also use these equations to get a good estimate. Just plug in the numbers and do the math:

For Men:
66 + (6.3 x weight in pounds) + (12.9 x height in inches) - (6.8 x age in years)

For Women:
655 + (4.3 x weight in pounds) + (4.7 x height in inches) - (4.7 x age in years)

For example, Jasmine is 42 years old, she is 5'3, and weighs 125 pounds. Here is how we figure out how many calories she should consume each day without any exercise:

655 + (4.3 x weight in pounds) + (4.7 x height in inches) - (4.7 x age in years)
655 + (4.3 x 125) + (4.7 x 63) − (4.7 x 42)
655 + (537.5) + (296.1) − (197.4)
1,291.2 calories per day

To lose weight, simply consume slightly less than your daily number of recommended calories. Keep in mind that this number is not factoring in your daily exercise, so however many calories you burn during exercise, you can add to the amount of calories you can eat.

Estimates of calories burned during exercise:

You can use Google or find an exercise application for your phone or tablet to find out how many calories different work-outs burn. However, the following chart shows about how many calories you will burn for various exercises based on your weight. You can use it to gauge the amount of calories you are burning during your daily activities.

Again, remember not to obsess over calories. You only want to have a rough idea of how many calories you are using each day to help build your meal plans.

If you have a consistent daily exercise routine, add those calories to your daily calorie intake. For example, if you completed the above equation, and you found that you should have 2,300 calories per day and you are burning 500 calories per day by exercise, then plan your meals according to a 2,800-calorie diet (2,300 + 500).

Exercise & Calories Burned per Hour	130 lbs	155 lbs	180 lbs	205 lbs
Aerobics, high impact	413	493	572	651
Aerobics, low impact	295	352	409	465
Basketball game, competitive	472	563	654	745
Basketball, shooting baskets	266	317	368	419
Bowling	177	211	245	279
Boxing, punching bag	354	422	490	558
Calisthenics, light, pushups, sit-ups	207	246	286	326
Calisthenics, fast, pushups, sit-ups	472	563	654	745
Canoeing, rowing, moderate	413	493	572	651
Circuit training, minimal rest	472	563	654	745
Cycling, <10mph, leisure bicycling	236	281	327	372
Gardening, general	236	281	327	372
General cleaning	207	246	286	326
Gymnastics	236	281	327	372
Hiking, cross-country	354	422	490	558
Housework, moderate	207	246	286	326
Judo, karate, jujitsu, martial arts	590	704	817	931
Kayaking	295	352	409	465
Mild stretching	148	176	204	233
Mowing lawn, walking, power mower	325	387	449	512
Rowing machine, moderate	413	493	572	651
Running, 6 mph (10 min mile)	590	704	817	931

Running, 7 mph (8.5 min mile) 679 809 940 1070
Stationary cycling, moderate 413 493 572 651
Stretching, hatha yoga 236 281 327 372
Swimming laps, freestyle, fast 590 704 817 931
Tai chi 236 281 327 372
Playing tennis 413 493 572 651
Walking/running, playing, moderate 236 281 327 372
Walking 3 mph, moderate 195 232 270 307
Weight-lifting, body-building, vigorous 354 422 490 558
Weight-lifting, light workout 177 211 245 279

Chapter 4: getting started: setting yourself up for success

When starting the DASH Diet, you should always prepare and plan ahead. Write out your meals for the week using the information and recipes provided in the upcoming chapters. Make adjuments based on your preferences, but keep in mind your daily servings of each food group. Once you have the meals mapped out, write up a grocery list and make sure have all the ingredients you need.

During Phase 1, the first two weeks of your DASH Diet journey, follow these guidelines to help set yourself up for changing your eating habits to adhere to the DASH Diet program.

- Eat an unlimited amount of non-starchy vegetables

- Eat as many dark and leafy greens as possible

- Be sure to get the right amounts of potassium (4,700 mg), calcium (1,250 mg), magnesium (500 mg), and fiber (30 g) every day

- Avoid foods that are high in carbohydrates like bread, pasta, potatoes, and rice

- Keep sodium intake below 2,300 mg per day

Once you finish Phase 1, the following guidelines will help keep you on track until the DASH Diet lifestyle becomes second nature to you.

- Cover your plate with colors to create variety

- Keep your intake of nutrients around 55% carbohydrates, 18% protein, and 27% fats (up to 6% saturated fats) of your calories

- Emphasize vegetables (especially dark, leafy greens), whole grains, fruits, low-fat dairy products, fish, and lean meats

- Treat vegetables as the main course and have at least two different ones

- Choose chicken and fish over red meat, and make sure all meats are lean

- Fish can be fatty because fish fat is good fat

- Be sure to choose low-fat or nonfat dairy options

- Have a small amount of nuts and seeds only 3 times per week

- Maintain the right amounts of potassium (4,700 mg), calcium (1,250 mg), magnesium (500 mg), and fiber (30 g) every day

- Choose sugar-free sweets whenever possible

- Gradually lower your sodium intake from 2,300 mg to 1,500 mg per day

- Prepare fruit-based desserts, instead of pastries or flour-based desserts

Brief Overview:
What to eat during Phase 1:
- Lots of non-starchy vegetables
- Leafy greens
- Low-Fat dairy
- Lean meats and poultry
- Fatty fish
- Nuts and seeds
- Avocado
- Sweeteners instead of sugar

What to eat during Phase 2:
- All of the above foods
- Fruits
- Whole grains

What NOT to eat:
- High salt foods
- High saturated fat foods
- High sugar foods

Know your serving sizes

Phase 1 foods and servings sizes

During phase 1, you will focus heavily on dark, leafy greens like spinach and broccoli. Every day you can have an unlimited amount of non-starchy vegetables; 2-4 servings of low-fat dairy; 5-11 ounces of lean meats, fish, or poultry; 1-4 servings of healthy fats; and 1-2 servings of nuts, beans, and seeds.

If you are consuming lower daily calories, you'll want to opt for the lower daily servings of dairy, healthy fats, and lean meats, fish, and poultry. If you are finding that your hunger is persistent, add more non-starchy vegetables to each meal.

Phase 2 foods servings sizes by daily calorie count

The following chart will help you determine how many serving sizes you should have each day based on your caloric intake. You should view this chart as a guide. It is certainly okay to round up or down serving sizes based on your needs and preferences.

Daily Calories	1600	1800	2000	2200	2400	2600	2800	3000
Grains	6	7	8	9	10	11	12	13
Vegetables	3	3	4	4	4.5	5	5	5.5
Fruits	4	4	4.5	5	5.5	6	6.5	7
Fat-free or lowfat dairy	2-3	2	2.5	2.5	3	3	3.5	3.5
Lean meats, poultry, and fish	4.5	5	6	6.5	7	7.5	8	8.5
Nuts, seeds, and legumes*	.5	.5	.5	.5	.5	1	1	1
Fats and oils	2	2	2.5	2.5	3	3	3.5	3.5
Sweets and added sugars**	.5	.5	.5	1	1	1	1	1

*With a 2000 calorie diet, nuts, seeds, and legumes are approximately 3 servings per week

**With a 2000 calorie diet, sweets and sugars are approximately 5 servings per week

Chapter 5: grocery list

The DASH Diet emphasizes vegetables, low-fat dairy products, and once you pass into phase 2, fruits and whole grains. It includes a healthy amount of legumes, lean meats, poultry and fish; and it allows a small amount of red meat, fats, and sweets. It is low in saturated fat, total fat, and cholesterol.

Food in the DASH Diet is broken down into categories just like the food pyramid or the Five Daily Food Groups. These food groups help you keep track of how well you are following the DASH Diet guidelines, based on the serving sizes for each group.

For example, based on a 2000 calorie diet in phase 1, every day you will have a minimum of 5 servings of non-starchy vegetables; 2-4 servings of low-fat or nonfat dairy; 2-4 serving of lean meats, fish, poultry, eggs; 1-4 servings of healthy fats; and 1-2 servings of nuts, beans, and seeds. A serving size of cooked lean meat, poultry, or fish is three ounces. A good reference is 3 ounces of meat is about the same size as a deck of cards.

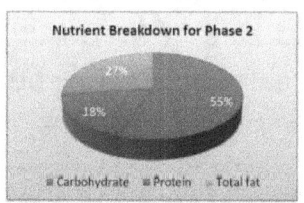

Based on a 2000 calorie diet in Phase 2, you will eat 6-8 servings of whole grains; 4-5 servings of vegetables; 4-5 servings of fruit; 2-3 servings of low-fat dairy; 6 servings of lean meats, poultry, or fish; and 2-3 servings of healthy fats every day. Additionally, each week you can have 4-5 servings of nuts, seeds, or beans and 5 or less servings of sugary sweets.

At first, following the DASH Diet takes some work, especially when you don't know what you should eat. Let's look at the DASH Diet food groups to get an idea of how to make delicious food recipes without getting bored.

Vegetables:

Once you are in Phase 2 of the DASH Diet, you can eat any vegetables. However, it is best to eat as many non-starchy vegetables as possible. Dark, green, leafy, vegetables are much more nutritious and low in calories. While starchy vegetables can make you feel full, they also tend to lead to more cravings. High fiber, non-starchy vegetables make you feel full without the cravings.

Many vegetables provide fiber, vitamins, and blood pressure-lowering minerals such as potassium and magnesium. Choose vegetables like broccoli, spinach, collard greens, and kale at first, but also eat plenty of sweet potatoes, carrots, green beans, green peas, lima beans, squash, sweet potatoes, or tomatoes.

One serving could be a half of a cup of raw or cooked vegetables, or a cup of raw, green, leafy vegetables.

Whole Grains:

Whole grains are good sources of energy, fiber, and nutrients. While the DASH Diet doesn't require that all grain servings be whole grain, it's best to choose whole grain whenever possible.

Whole grains include foods such as brown rice, whole wheat or multigrain breads, whole wheat pasta, oats, quinoa, barley, and buckwheat. You can also choose from foods such as oatmeal, cereals, English muffins, pita bread, bagels, grits, and snacks like unsalted pretzels and popcorn.

One serving of whole grains could be a slice of whole wheat bread or a half cup of cooked pasta or rice.

Fruits:

Many fruits are high in fiber, potassium, magnesium, and other vitamins and minerals. They are also typically low in fat. Choose from a wide variety of fruits including apples, apricots, bananas, pears, dates, grapes, oranges, grapefruit, mangoes, melons, peaches, pineapples, raisins, strawberries, and blueberries.

One serving may include a half of a cup of fresh or frozen fruit, or a half glass of juice.

Lean Meats, Poultry, and Fish:

Meats are rich in proteins, B vitamins, zinc, and other nutrients. However, DASH dieters should limit their meat consumption and eat mostly fruits and vegetables. Whenever possible, choose meat and eggs that are grass-fed or organic. This helps to minimize any bacteria and steroid hormone intake.

Always select lean meats and trim away visible fat. When eating poultry, remove skin. The key is to avoid fats from meat and poultry as much as possible; however, you should try to eat fatty fish often. Fatty fish such as salmon, herring, and tuna are high in heart-healthy omega-3 fatty acids; so when you choose fatty fish, eat the fats. Cook lean meats, poultry, and fish by broiling, roasting, poaching, or grilling.

One serving of lean meat, poultry, or fish equals 1 ounce. 3 ounces is about the size of a deck of cards; so when you eat a deck of cards-sized piece, that equals 3 of your servings.

Meat: Lean meat options can include beef, veal, goat, lamb, and others, but you have to select the lean versions.

Poultry: You can choose from chicken, duck, quail, and others, but try to find free range or organic.

Fish: Prioritize anything that is caught wild like salmon, mackerel, catfish, tuna, mahi-mahi, flounder, cod, halibut, snapper, and trout. You can also choose from shellfish such as, crab, mussels, oysters, lobster, clams, squid, and scallops.

One serving may include 1 ounce of cooked, skinless poultry, lean meat or seafood, or 1 ounce of tuna, packed in water, with no salt added.

Dairy Products:

Dairy products are major sources of calcium, protein, and vitamin D. It is best if you choose either low-fat or fat-free. You can choose a variety of dairy products, but more often you should try fat-free or skim milk; fat-free, low-fat, or reduced-fat cheese; or fat- free or low-fat yogurt.

One serving could include 1 cup of skim milk, or milk that is 1 percent fat, 1.5 ounces of cheese, or 1 cup of yogurt.

Fats and Oils:

The body needs fat to properly absorb essential vitamins and other nutrients, and it needs healthy fats to help maintain the immune system. The trick here is to get the right type of fat and the right amount. While on the DASH Diet, fat should be about 28 percent of calories, and the priority should be monounsaturated fats.

Saturated Fats: These fats are considered unhealthy and should be less than 6% of your daily calories.

Monounsaturated Fats and Polyunsaturated Fats: Monounsaturated fats can help lower your cholesterol levels when you eat them in place of saturated or trans fats. They also keep your heart rhythm normal, reduce inflammation, and help regulate your insulin and blood sugar levels. Monounsaturated fats are found in liquid oils such as olive, canola, peanut, safflower, and sunflower oils. Avocados are rich in monounsaturated fats too.

Polyunsaturated fats can also help lower bad cholesterol levels when you eat them instead of saturated or trans fats. They might also boost good cholesterol levels. For example, omega-3 fatty acid is good for your heart and helps reduce high blood pressure.
Polyunsaturated fats are found in soybean, corn, and flax oil, but also in fatty fish, such as salmon, mackerel, and trout.

Nuts, Seeds, and Legumes:

Nuts, seeds, and legumes are good sources of protein, potassium, magnesium, fiber, and other essential nutrients. Soybean products, like tofu, are good protein sources.

You can choose from a wide variety of nuts, seeds, and legumes; but eat from this group sparingly, because serving sizes are small and you should only have 4-5 servings per week.

Examples from this food group include sunflower seeds, almonds, peanuts, pistachios, kidney beans, lentils, and split peas.

Sweets:

The DASH Diet does not eliminate sweets for your food plan, but it does limit them. The plan recommends having 5 or less servings of sweets per week.

You should aim for sweets that are low in fat like fruit-flavored gelatin, sorbet, hard candy, jelly, or maple syrup. You can choose fruit options to satisfy any additional cravings for sweets without having servings from the sweets category. Also, try sugar substitutes whenever possible.

One serving could include 1 cup of soda, a half of a cup of sorbet, or 1 tablespoon of sugar, jam, or jelly.

Alcohol:

The DASH diet recommends no more than two alcoholic drinks for men and one for women each day.

Chapter 6: dash diet: the essentials

One of the best things about the DASH Diet, and why so many people succeed by following it, is that it is a simple strategy. Rather than a restrictive diet with complicated science, the DASH Diet is a healthy food and nutrition plan, that allows a wide variety of food choices.

While it helps to know the numbers (calories, serving size, etc.), if you keep the guidelines in mind, the DASH Diet will come easy to you, and the numbers will just be a tool to help you reach perfection. Here is a simple review of everything we learned so far:

Eat your vegtables:

Vegetables are going to be your go to food as much as possible. They will provide you fiber to make you feel full and nutrients to keep your body working its best. If you prefer meat or breads, enjoy them and make sure you add a couple vegetable sides.

Maintain low sodium intake:
The DASH Diet does not eliminate certain foods or food groups. Instead, it recommends decreasing foods that are high in sodium and saturated fat, and increasing low or no sodium foods.
Follow the serving sizes:

Serving sizes are what make the DASH Diet so easy. With a little preparation you can use your daily calories numbers to determine your serving size for each food group. Once you know how many servings of each food group you should have daily, it's as easy as picking the right number of foods from each group.

Embrace variety:

DASH Diet stresses food variety to ensure a nutrient-rich diet. Given the focus on lowering blood pressure, it prioritizes nutrients that help reduce blood pressure such as potassium, calcium, and magnesium.
Read the labels:

Read the nutrition labels on foods to compare the amount of sodium in products. Look for the sodium content in milligrams and the Percent Daily Value. Aim for foods that have less than 5 percent of the Daily Value of sodium, but also make sure you don't eat more sodium than your recommended daily amount. Additionally, you want to read the label to check your protein, carbohydrate, and fat intake, as well as vitamin intake.

When purchasing any packaged food, be sure to read the labels. This can be a lot of work at first, but if you keep track of which products fulfill your dietary needs, within a short time you will be simply writing up a grocery list and purchasing the products you know are good.

When searching for the best food products, it will help to understand some basic terminology. Here is a simple breakdown for sodium and fat content:

Sodium

Sodium free or salt free = Less than 5 mg per serving
Very low sodium = 35 mg or less of sodium per serving
Low sodium = 140 mg or less of sodium per serving
Reduced or less sodium = At least 25 percent less sodium than the regular version

Light in sodium = 50 percent less sodium than the regular version

Unsalted or no salt added = No salt added to the food, but the food might still be high in sodium

Fat

Fat-free = Less than 0.5 g per serving

Low saturated fat = 1 g or less per serving and 15 percent or less of calories from saturated fat

Low-fat = 3 g or less per serving

Reduced fat = At least 25 percent less fat than the regular version

Light in fat = Half the fat compared to the regular version

Exercise daily:

Exercise is essential for a healthy lifestyle. If you want to get the best results from the DASH Diet, then be sure to exercise for at least 20-30 minutes each day. Exercise isn't just a way to lose weight; it helps the body function properly and increases overall health. Even simply walking a lot can help regulate weight loss and blood sugar levels.

Get your nutrients:

Do your best to get plan meals that give you the proper nutritional breakdown every day. The chart below highlights some of the main nutrients that you will want to focus on while you get used to the DASH Diet.

Nutritional Breakdown for Phase 2 (based on a 2000-calorie diet):

Total fat	27% of calories
Saturated fat	6% of calories
Protein	18% of calories
Carbohydrate	55% of calories
Cholesterol	150 mg
Sodium	2,300 or 1,500 mg

Potassium	*4,700 mg*
Calcium	*1,250 mg*
Magnesium	*500 mg*
Fiber	*30 g*

Chapter 7: let's get started step-by-step

Part 1: Starting the DASH Diet

Step 1. First talk to your doctor to ensure there are no health risks for you in starting the diet, especially if you have any medical conditions

Step 2. Determine your recommended daily calories and how many calories you burn in your regular exercise routines

Step 3. Determine how many servings you can consume daily from each food group

Step 4. Plan you meals for a full week, make a grocery list, and go shopping

Part 2: Start your two-week, Phase 1 program

Step 5. Consume as many non-starchy vegetables as you like during breakfast, lunch, and dinner

Step 6. Consume 2-4 servings of low-fat or nonfat dairy, and 5-11 ounces of lean meats, fish, poultry, or eggs per day

Step 7. Consume healthy fats

Step 8. Don't stress too much about calorie intake

Step 9. Exercise daily for at least 20-30 minutes

Step 10. Consume less than 2,300 mg of sodium per day

Part 3: Transition to Phase 2, your lifelong DASH Diet

Step 11. Gradually add servings of whole grains and fruits to your daily meal plan

Step 12. Gradually decrease your daily sodium intake from 2,300 mg to 1,500 mg

Step 13. Assess how your health has improved, and if you feel it has not, re-evaluate your plan and make sure you are correctly following the DASH Diet

Step 14. Celebrate and enjoy your new health lifestyle!

Chapter 8: phase 1 meal plan

Here is a sample meal phase 1 of the DASH Diet. You can follow this for two weeks and then begin to add your whole grain and fruit servings to move into phase 2.

While following the meal plan below, be sure to add sides of vegetables with your meals to help curb hunger and cravings. You can also have sugar free juices, low sodium vegetable juices with meals, and sugar free Jell-O for desserts. Finally, you should have snacks between meals. Looking for low fat cheese sticks or baby carrots for easy options. Just be sure to read labels and make a plan where you consume the correct number of calories and serving sizes from each food group.

DAY	BREAKFAST	LUNCH	DINNER
Day 1	Breakfast Scramble	Chicken Salad Salad	Walnut Crusted Salmon
Day 2	Hard Boiled	Spinach	Sesame-Maple

	Eggs	Avocado Salad	Roasted Tofu
Day 3	Poached Eggs with Avocado and Tomato	Collard Green Leaf Chicken Wrap	Romaine Leaf Fish Tacos
Day 4	Hard Boiled Eggs	Tuna Salad	Crispy Tofu Blend
Day 5	Spinach and Feta Omelet	Grilled Chicken and Pine Nuts Salad	Veg Kebabs
Day 6	Mushroom and Onion Quiches	Collard Green Turkey Wrap	Breadless Turkey Burgers
Day 7	Shakshuka	Italian Eggplant and Tomatoes	Chicken Stir Fry

Chapter 9: dash diet recipes

Breakfast Recipes

Recipe 1: Breakfast Scramble

Ingredients
2 large eggs
½ cup chopped tomato
¼ cup chopped green pepper
¼ cup chopped onions
1/8 teaspoon black pepper
1/8 teaspoon hot sauce
1 teaspoon of fresh, chopped cilantro

Directions
1. Cover the pan with cooking spray; heat on medium-high until hot
2. Scramble eggs in a bowl
3. Add bell pepper, and onions; sauté until slightly brown, then add tomatoes and reduce heat to low
4. Add eggs, black pepper, and hot sauce, and stir until eggs are set but still moist
5. Remove from heat add cilantro

Recipe 2: Poached Eggs with Avocado and Tomato

Ingredients
2 eggs
½ an avocado thickly sliced
½ a tomato thickly sliced
2 tablespoons grated Parmesan cheese
¼ teaspoon of black pepper
Fresh basil and thyme chopped

Directions

1. Lay tomato and avocado slices on the plate
2. Bring a pot of water to boil
3. Crack the eggs directly into the boiling water, turn down the heat to medium for 2 minutes then take off the element.
4. When eggs are finished cooking, remove them from the water with a slotted spoon, and lay the eggs on top of the tomato and avocado slice
5. Sprinkle Parmesan cheese, pepper, basil, and thyme on top of the eggs

Recipe 3: Spinach and Feta Omelet

Ingredients
2 Eggs
2 chopped garlic cloves
½ teaspoon of cilantro
½ teaspoon cayenne pepper
¼ cup Feta cheese
1 large handful of chopped spinach

Directions
1. Cover the pan with cooking spray; heat on medium-high until hot
2. Scramble eggs in a bowl
3. Add the garlic cloves to the pan and let brown
4. Add eggs and stir gently while they begin to cook and add the cayenne pepper and once the eggs are almost finished cooking, add the spinach
5. Cover the pan and cook for 30 to 60 seconds more
6. Sprinkle with Feta cheese and fresh ground pepper
7. Top with a little cilantro and serve

Recipe 4: Mushroom and Onion Quiches

Ingredients

5 eggs
3 egg whites
1 cup 1% milk
1 teaspoon extra-virgin olive oil
8 ounces sliced mushrooms
1/4 cup of chopped white onions
1/4 cup shredded Swiss cheese
1 teaspoon black pepper
1 teaspoon of thyme

Directions
1. Preheat to 325 degrees F.
2. Coat a nonstick muffin tin generously with cooking spray
3. Heat a large nonstick skillet over medium-high heat. Add onion and cook until golden brown add mushrooms and thyme. Stir until brown.
4. Transfer the blend to a bowl and let cool
5. Add cheese and pepper.
6. Whisk eggs, egg whites and milk in a medium bowl. Divide the egg mixture evenly among the prepared muffin cups.
7. Add a big spoon of the blend into each cup.
8. Bake until the tops are just beginning to brown, 25 minutes.

9. Let cool for 5 minutes. Then flip the pan over to remove the quiches

Recipe 5: Shakshuka (Middle Eastern Eggs and Tomato)

Ingredients
6 eggs
1 tablespoon extra virgin olive oil
1/2 medium onion, diced
1 clove garlic minced
1 medium green or red bell pepper, chopped
4 cups ripe diced tomatoes,
2 tablespoon tomato paste
1 teaspoon chili powder, mild
1 teaspoon cumin
1 teaspoon paprika
1/8 teaspoon cayenne pepper
1/8 teaspoon black pepper

Directions
1. Heat a large skillet on medium.
2. Add olive oil in the pan. Add chopped onion, sauté for a few minutes until the onion begins to soften. Add garlic and continue to sauté
3. Add the bell pepper, sauté for 5 minutes until softened.
4. Add tomatoes and tomato paste to pan, stir until blended. Add spices and stir
5. Allow mixture to simmer for 5-7 minutes until it starts to reduce.

6.Crack the eggs, one at a time, directly over the tomato mixture, making sure to space them evenly over the sauce.

7.Allow the eggs to cook in the sauce until they are slightly runny

Lunch recipes

Recipe 6: Chicken Salad Salad

Ingredients

1/3 cup chopped or shredded cooked chicken or turkey
2 tablespoons chopped celery
1 tablespoon light mayonnaise
1 tablespoon salsa
1 tablespoon shredded cheddar cheese
1 cup of baby spinach

Directions
1. In a bowl combine chicken, celery, mayonnaise, salsa, and cheese; and stir
2. Scoop chicken salad on to a bed of raw spinach

Recipe 7: Spinach and Avocado Salad

Ingredients

1 cup of baby spinach
1/2 small avocado peeled and chopped
¼ of red onion chopped
1 tablespoons balsamic vinegar
1/2 teaspoons of olive oil
1/2 teaspoons toasted sesame seeds

1/4 teaspoon black pepper

Directions

1. Mixed toasted sesame seeds with balsamic vinegar and olive oil
2. Lay spinach on a plate and top with avocado and red onion
3. Drizzle balsamic dressing over salad

Recipe 8: Collard Green Leaf Chicken Wrap

Ingredients
½ cup chopped cooked chicken breast
1 large collard green leaf
½ cup of chopped spinach
3 tablespoons chopped cherry tomatoes
2 tablespoons chopped red onions
2 tablespoons chopped celery
1 tablespoon 2% Pepper Jack Cheese
½ teaspoon of olive oil

Preparation
1. Heat pan on medium-low
2. Add olive oil and warm collard green leaf on both sides until it becomes soft
3. Mix chopped ingredients with chicken
4. Spoon into open collard green leaf, fold in the sides, and roll

Recipe 9: Tuna Salad

Ingredients
1 can water packed, low sodium tuna
2 hard boiled egg, diced
1 cup romaine lettuce
2 tablespoons of grated carrot
8 grape tomatoes cut in half,
1/8 cup of shredded red cabbage
1/4 cup diced celery
½ cup light mayonnaise
1 teaspoon mustard
1/8 teaspoon of black pepper
1/8 teaspoon of cayenne pepper

Directions
1. Drain tuna and mix together with egg, celery, mustard and mayonnaise.
2. Season with black pepper and cayenne pepper
3. Make salad base with romaine lettuce, topped tomato, carrots, and red cabbage
4. Place 1/2 cup tuna on top

Recipe 10: Grilled Chicken and Pine Nut Salad

Ingredients

3 ounces of grilled chicken breast
2 ounces mixed greens
1 ounces of roasted pine nuts
4 teaspoons of vinaigrette dressing
1 tablespoon of Parmesan cheese

Preparation Method

1.Mix greens, pine nuts and vinaigrette dressing
2.Slice grilled chicken and lay it over salad
3.Top with Parmesean cheese

Recipe 11: Italian Eggplant and Tomato

Ingredients

1 large eggplant pealed and cubed
1 cup of chopped tomato
2 cloves garlic, minced
1 tablespoon of olive oil
1 teaspoon of oregano
1 teaspoon of thyme
1 teaspoon of rosemary
1/2 cup chopped fresh cilantro

Directions
1. In medium pan, warm olive oil on medium-high heat. Add eggplant and sauté 1 minute. Add garlic and sauté 30 seconds.
2. Reduce heat to low and cover pan; let cook for about 10 minutes until the eggplant is soft.
3. Stir in oregano, thyme, and rosemary, and let cook for 30 seconds
4. Stir in tomatoes and bring to a boil.
5. Reduce heat to medium-low and cook for about 7 more minutes.

Dinner recipes

Recipe 12: Walnut Crusted Salmon

Ingredients

1.2 lb Salmon fillets
1 ounces of walnut
2 teaspoons of honey
½ teaspoon Dijon mustard
¼ teaspoon dill
1 tablespoon ghee 1
1/8 teaspoon black pepper

Directions

1. Preheat the oven to 350F. Add walnuts, honey, your spices and mustard in food processor and make a paste
2. Heat the pan and add ghee and fry dry salmon fillets for about 3 minutes
3. Add the walnut paste to the top side of salmon fillets
4. Once they seared, transfer them to an oven and bake for about 8 -10 minutes

Recipe 12: Sesame-Maple Roasted Tofu

Ingredients

14-ounce firm tofu cut into cubes
1 medium red onion, sliced
3 cups sugar snap peas, trimmed
1 tablespoon sesame seeds
1 tablespoon tahini
1 tablespoon low-sodium soy sauce
2 teaspoons canola oil
2 teaspoons toasted sesame oil
2 teaspoons pure maple syrup
1 teaspoon cider vinegar
1/4 teaspoon freshly ground pepper

Directions
1. Preheat oven to 450 degrees F
2. Mix tahini, soy sauce, maple syrup and vinegar in a small dish
3. Toss tofu, onion, canola oil, sesame oil, salt and pepper in a large bowl then spread on a large baking sheet and roast for about 15 minutes until the tofu is lightly golden on top and the onions brown
4. Remove the tofu from the oven, add snap peas and drizzle with the maple sauce
5. Sprinkle with sesame seeds.

6. Return to the oven and continue roasting for about 10 minute until the snap peas are crisp

Recipe 13: Romaine Leaf Fish Taco

Ingredients

1/2 pound tilapia fillets
1/2 cup reduced fat sour cream
½ cup of salsa
1 teaspoon ground cumin
1 tablespoon Canola Oil
2 tablespoons of shredded mozzarella cheese
6 Romain lettuce leaves

Directions
1. Stir together sour cream and salsa
2. Sprinkle fish with cumin
3. Heat oil in large nonstick skillet over medium-high heat then place fish in skillet
4. Cook 3 to 4 minutes on each side or until fish flakes easily with fork
5. Separate fish into 6 pieces. Place 1 piece on each leaf, top with sour cream, salsa, and cheese

Recipe 14: Crispy Tofu Blend

Ingredients

14-ounce firm tofu cut into cubes
2 cups fresh sugar snap peas
3 tablespoons of low-sodium soy sauce
1/4 cup yellow cornmeal
1/8 teaspoon ground red pepper
2 teaspoons toasted sesame oil
1 medium red sweet pepper, cut into thin strips
1 medium yellow sweet pepper, cut into thin strips
8 green onions cut into 2-inch pieces
2 teaspoons olive oil
1 tablespoon toasted sesame seed

Directions

1. Lay tofu cubes in a baking dish and pour 2 tablespoons of the soy sauce over tofu
2. Let stand at room temperature for 15 minutes, then drain
3. In a shallow dish combine cornmeal and ground red pepper.
4. Carefully dip tofu slices in cornmeal mixture; press gently to coat both sides.

5. Pour 1 teaspoon of the sesame oil into a large nonstick skillet. Preheat over medium-high heat. Stir-fry sweet pepper strips for 2 minutes.

6. Add pea pods and green onions; stir-fry for 2 to 3 minutes until crisp-tender.

7. Remove skillet from heat; stir in the remaining 1 tablespoon teriyaki sauce.

8. In a different pan, heat the remaining 1 teaspoon sesame oil and the cooking oil over medium heat.

9. Cook the coated tofu slices for 2 to 3 minutes on each side or until crisp and golden brown, using a spatula to turn carefully.

10. Place tofu slices over vegetable mixture and sprinkle with sesame seeds

Recipe 15: Veg-Kebabs

Ingredients

8 cherry tomatoes
8 button mushrooms
1 small zucchini, sliced into 8 pieces
1 red onion, cut into 4 wedges
1 green bell pepper, seeded and cut into 4 pieces
1 red bell pepper, seeded and cut into 4 pieces
1/2 cup fat-free Italian dressing
1/2 cup brown rice
1 cup water
4 wooden skewers, soaked in water for 30 minutes, or metal skewers

Directions
1. Place the tomatoes, mushrooms, zucchini, onion and peppers in a sealed plastic bag. Add the Italian dressing and shake to coat the vegetables evenly. Marinate the vegetables for at least 10 minutes.
2. Prior to lighting, lightly coat grill with nonstick cooking spray. If using the broiler, you can lay kebabs on tin foil
3. Preheat grill a hot or broiler.
4. Thread 2 tomatoes, 2 mushrooms, 2 zucchini slices, 1 onion wedge, and 1 green and red pepper slice onto each skewer. Place the kebabs on the grill rack or broiler pan. Baste with leftover marinade.

5.Grill or broil the kebabs, turning as needed, until the vegetables are tender, about 5 to 8 minutes.

www.ingramcontent.com/pod-product-compliance
Lightning Source LLC
Chambersburg PA
CBHW071436070526
44578CB00001B/107